W

KV-579-243

The seven
deadly
sins of

Obesity

The seven deadly sins of

Obesity

How the modern world is making us fat

edited by **JANE DIXON** *and*
DOROTHY H BROOM

UNSW PRESS

A UNSW Press book

Published by
University of New South Wales Press Ltd
University of New South Wales
Sydney NSW 2052
AUSTRALIA
www.unswpress.com.au

© UNSW Press 2007
First published 2007

This book is copyright. Apart from any fair dealing for the purpose of private study, research, criticism or review, as permitted under the Copyright Act, no part may be reproduced by any process without written permission. While copyright of the work as a whole is vested in UNSW Press, copyright of individual chapters is retained by the chapter authors. Inquiries should be addressed to the publisher.

National Library of Australia
Cataloguing-in-Publication entry
    The seven deadly sins of obesity: how the modern world is
    making us fat.
    Includes index.
    ISBN 978086840 9559.
    1. Obesity - Australia - Social aspects. 2. Lifestyles - Australia - Health aspects.
    3. Well-being - Australia. I. Dixon, Jane, 1951- . II. Broom, Dorothy H.
    363.810994

Design Di Quick
Cover photo Karen Mork
Printer Griffin Press

The editors acknowledge with gratitude that ARC Discovery Project DP0559439 supplied some of the research support for this book. They also are thankful to the Australian National University Publications Committee for a small subsidy to assist in the book's publication.

CONTENTS

CONTRIBUTORS

Cathy Banwell has a background in social anthropology and public health. She has an ongoing interest in the sociocultural trends and environments behind the consumption practices around food, alcohol and other drugs and their negative health consequences. She is a research fellow at the National Centre for Epidemiology and Population Health (NCEPH), Australian National University, Canberra, Australia. cathy.banwell@anu.edu.au

Dorothy Broom is a sociologist and senior fellow at NCEPH. Before her current appointment she was convenor of the ANU's Women's Studies Program. She has spent more than 30 years teaching and studying gender and other aspects of the sociology of health and illness. In 1991, she published *Damned If We Do: Contradictions in Women's Health Care* (Allen & Unwin), a political history of Australia's feminist community health centres. dorothy.broom@anu.edu.au

Richard Denniss is strategic advisor to the Australian Greens. Richard is an economist with a particular interest in the role of regulation in a modern economy. He has previously worked as deputy director of The Australia Institute, was chief of staff to the then leader of the Australian Democrats, Senator Natasha Stott Despoja, and has lectured in economics at the University of Newcastle. Richard.Denniss@aph.gov.au

Jane Dixon is a sociologist whose research focuses on transformations in food systems and culinary cultures and how these transformations are having an impact on obesity and other public health issues. Her book *The Changing Chicken: Chooks, Cooks and Culinary Culture* was published by UNSW Press in 2002. She is a fellow at NCEPH. jane.dixon@anu.edu.au

Anni Dugdale is a senior lecturer in the School of Business & Government at University of Canberra. Her research focuses on the mutual co-construction of technology and society. Anni.Dugdale@Canberra.edu.au

Sharon Friel is an epidemiologist and is currently the principal research fellow for the secretariat of the WHO Commission on Social Determinants of Health, based at the International Institute for Society and Health, University College London. She is also a Vincent Fairfax Family Foundation fellow, part-time, at NCEPH. Much of her work is concerned with research, policy and practice in matters relating to international and national level social determinants of inequalities in diet and health. sharon.friel@anu.edu.au

Sarah Hinde has spent the last few years examining the social, cultural and economic aspects of car reliance, and studying the relationship between Australia's transport system, class inequalities and population health. Sarah is working towards a PhD at NCEPH, ANU. sarah.hinde@anu.edu.au

Megan Shipley is a project manager at NCEPH. She currently works on Health for Life!, a project examining the impact of work on families' psychological, emotional and physical wellbeing. Megan has a background in psychology. Megan.Shipley@anu.edu.au

Julie Smith is an Australian Research Council postdoctoral fellow, the Australian Centre for Economic Research on Health,

College of Medicine and Health Sciences, Australian National University. Formerly a senior economist in Australian and New Zealand treasuries, she has authored two books on tax policy, and published on public finance and health issues in journals across several disciplines, including on the economic value of mothers milk. Julie.smith@anu.edu.au

Lyndall Strazdins is a research fellow at NCEPH. Her research and publications have focused on contemporary work and family life, including: work at unsociable times and parent and child wellbeing; employed mothers, time pressure and musculoskeletal pain; job insecurity and adult mental health; and the impact of high job quality (jobs with autonomy, security, flexibility and family friendly provisions) on parent wellbeing, family functioning and children. lyndall.strazdins@anu.edu.au

Christine Winter is a historian who was employed on the ARC funded Weight of Modernity project in 2005. Currently she is a researcher with the Official History of Australian Peacekeeping and Post-Cold War Operations, a joint project of the Australian War Memorial and the Strategic and Defence Studies Centre, ANU. Her latest projects are an exploration of National Socialism in Australasia, and a re-evaluation of impartial humanitarianism in the 20th century. Christine.Winter@anu.edu.au

PREFACE

While there is an overall consensus that fighting obesity is a high public health priority, this book appears within a highly charged context of claim and counterclaim as to the nature of the obesity problem. Is it a concern because of the evidence that obesity is a risk factor for premature death and disability? Is it a problem for the public health field because there is so much conflicting evidence as to the health significance of being clinically overweight and obese? Is obesity a benign health issue but a classical social problem because of its capacity to galvanise public opinion and provoke social divisions? Is it an economic and political problem because obesity simultaneously costs the government money (for health care and lost productivity) while fuelling economic growth through the production and distribution of goods and services to meet the needs of obese individuals? Is it an issue of aesthetics, where slim bodies are seen as more pleasing than fat bodies? Or is it simply the most recent in a long line of risk discourses following terrorism, drug taking, the gender wars, the Cold War and class conflict? Is a metaphorical War on Obesity being waged? The Australian government has an official 'Tough on Drugs' policy, but does it also have an unofficial 'Tough on Obesity' policy?

Debates about the nature of the problem raise a related issue: Should there be action, and if so, who should act? Some commentators insist that obesity is a social issue demanding political attention, while others judge it to be the province of the individual and a private matter. There are those who argue that the solution lies in industry self-regulation, while others question industry's capacity to self-regulate and instead call on government to restrict commercial activities, particularly in relation to the marketing and promotion of unhealthy foods and leisure activities. Australian governments are resisting such calls, and instead are asking parents to take responsibility. We note that these polarising discourses assign governments and individuals alike to ineffectual solutions.

This book contends that it is not helpful to play the game of 'pass the parcel' of responsibility. Instead of viewing individuals as sinful and riddled with vices (particularly sloth and gluttony), we argue that it is more appropriate to view contemporary social and physical environments as lacking the virtues necessary for people to adopt and maintain healthy behaviours. Our focus is on the environmental determinants of the rise in obesity.

Our selection of what constitutes an environmental sin arises from research conducted by a team at the National Centre for Epidemiology and Population Health (NCEPH) in 2003. In response to a question about 'the major social trends behind the rise in obesity in Australia in the last 50 years', 50 Australian experts in obesity and related fields agreed on seven explanations for changes in physical activity and food consumption patterns (the research is explained in the introduction).

We have recast the seven 'obesogenic' trends nominated by the experts as seven sins of modern environments, namely:

- The commodified environment
- The harried environment
- The pressured parenting environment
- The technological environment

- The car-reliant environment
- The marketed environment
- The environment of competing authorities.

We argue that they combine to generate significant detrimental impacts for health, including the rising prevalence of obesity. The implication of the chapters in this book is that if modern societies are to act to prevent further increases in obesity, they will have to intervene to alter the dynamics within social, economic, cultural and physical environments.

INTRODUCTION

Seven modern environmental sins of obesity

Dorothy H Broom and Jane Dixon

Background

Australians are getting fatter. Over half of adult Australians are overweight or obese, a proportion that has risen sharply in the last 20 years, with repercussions for the national economy and for the individuals concerned (Dixon & Waters, 2003). However, as Australian governments are devising their responses, responsibility for this latest 'epidemic' is being contested. Questions have been raised about whether governments ought to intervene in what some see as a private matter. When Australia's Governor-General Jeffreys publicly commented on the 'fat lifestyle' of Australian children, he exhorted parents to take greater control of their children's eating habits and physical activity (Vermeer, 2004). And in defending advertising food to children, the former chair of the Australian Broadcasting Association asserted: 'it is surely not the role of legislatures to forbid everything that people do legally but which may not be good for them ... the solution is ... to put a countervailing idea into the marketplace. In this case [obesity], arguments for exercise and good nutrition' (Flint, 2003).

In the meantime, consumers are finding that the marketplace offers everything but the solution. While corporate lawyers are preparing to defend their commercial clients against class actions from fat customers, increasing numbers of people join weight loss programs. Many people spend considerable sums on gyms and diets in order to lose weight, but others join size acceptance organisations to receive social support in the face of the marketplace onslaught and to cope with the significant stresses that accompany social pressure to conform to particular body stereotypes (www.naafa.org; www.bella.co.nz).

By contrast to the advocates of market-based solutions, some economic historians suggest that obesity is a disease of modernisation: the inevitable and unintended consequence of a particular form of economic development (Cutler et al., 2003). Typically, post-industrial capitalism ushers in a transition from communicable diseases to chronic conditions because it brings affluence, longevity and new health-damaging behaviours such as smoking, inactivity and over-nutrition. Australia exemplifies the circumstances that give rise to diseases of modernity, most of which are more prevalent and have worse health outcomes among people who are socially disadvantaged.

The emergence of a fatter society has taken place in a relatively short time and with a reversal in those most at risk. A century ago, an ample figure was associated with male privilege and female fecundity. The transitions in overweight from upper to lower classes indicate the operation of a complex interaction between changing social conditions and individual actions (Stearns, 1997). Certainly, genetic theories are not sufficient to explain the rapidity of change in the last 30 years or the differences between socioeconomic groups (McMichael, 2001).

The World Health Organization (WHO) has ranked obesity as one of ten preventable conditions that require urgent attention, but even this assessment has provoked dissent. In 2003, the WHO and the Food and Agriculture Organization issued a report containing guidelines to improve world nutrition and prevent chronic diseases. In particular, the report recommended that people limit their intake of sugars to no more than 10 per cent of total calories, drawing a hostile response from the sugar producers and processed food industry (Chopra & Darnton-Hill, 2004; Jain, 2004). Despite the debates, Australian governments have recognised obesity as an epidemic and a social problem, and the Federal government has included it as a National Research Priority. The peak medical research body, the National Health and Medical Research Council (NHMRC), has issued clinical guidelines for doctors to follow when treating overweight and obese patients (National Health and Medical Research Council, 2003). Obesity is rated as the fourth most important preventable health risk factor, accounting for just over 4 per cent of the burden of ill-health in Australia (Stephenson et al., 2000); and according to the National Obesity Taskforce (NOT), the economic costs attributable to this avoidable condition are already $1.3 billion a year (National Obesity Taskforce, 2003).

In an attempt to explain the epidemiologic evidence, the public health field is emphasising the contribution of the social context to collective weight gain. This perspective highlights the role of the physical, cultural and social environments of industrialised countries in encouraging a positive energy balance in the population. Swinburn and colleagues (1999) have characterised contemporary environments as 'obesogenic'; that is, they offer an abundance of high energy foods, sedentary jobs and leisure activities, and labour saving devices. While the general tenor of this research shifts the burden of responsibility away from individuals, it fuels a media-generated miasma, where people fear that they will drown 'in the rising ocean levels' of fat (Lambert, 2004, p. 99).

For some, the media's hysterical tones and the more general fixation with thinness are the real disease. In a best selling book, *The Obesity Myth: Why America's Obsession with Weight is Hazardous to Your Health*, Campos puts the case that obesity is rarely a health hazard and that pharmaceutical and diet industries have perpetrated a giant fraud upon the population (Campos, 2004). Paul Campos, a professor of law, argues that there is no health epidemic; rather, Americans inhabit a diet-distorting culture fostered by industry and by social elites who project their anxieties about over-consumption and race (African-Americans are significantly heavier than Anglo-Americans) onto the whole population. Having 'exposed' the fraud, he proceeds to counsel people to watch what they eat and to exercise regularly.

Campos builds this case on his evidence-based assessment that obesity does not do mortal harm. However, his view is not shared by many in the medical profession. A recent study in the *New England Medical Journal* reported that as the prevalence of childhood obesity grows, the current generation of children may 'live less healthful and shorter lives than their parents' (Olshansky, 2005). The researchers estimated that by 2050, the obese will lose two to five years of life expectancy because they will have carried the burden of extra weight for many more years than their parents. For the first time in American history, economic progress may not be accompanied by longer life expectancy. This trend may also be taking hold in Australia. After two decades of major advances in tackling Australia's biggest killer, coronary heart disease (CHD), the improvements have stalled and for some sub-populations the rates of CHD are again increasing (Humphreys & Dixon, 2004). The most plausible explanation is the rise in obesity, which is known to contribute to CHD, particularly if the weight is carried around the abdomen. Thus, while obesity does not kill outright, premature death may result from the complications that accompany obesity.

While we agree with a part of the Campos thesis, namely that prevailing social elite and medical cultures promote unhealthy bodily obsessions, we come to very different conclusions about what is needed to counteract the cultural influences. Unlike his rather simplistic notion that individuals can resist the environment's temptations by being more disciplined or by ignoring all that surrounds them, we argue for an environmental change strategy to shift obesity trends from their current potentially lethal trajectory.

The magnitude of the problem

In recent years, Australians have been bombarded with statistics about the nation's expanding waistline. Instead of exhaustively rehearsing the data, we provide only a few headline statistics, and propose standard arguments from public health about why obesity is worthy of societal attention. The chapter 'Unequal society, unhealthy weight' explores in greater detail the unequal distribution of obesity. That chapter shows obese people to be over-represented in low socioeconomic areas, in rural areas and among those on low incomes and with less education.

In the last 20 years, obesity prevalence has increased two and half times in Australia (Cameron et al., 2003). Two in three men and one in two women are overweight or obese, resulting in around 7.5 million Australians aged 25 years and over being of clinical concern (Dixon & Waters, 2003).

Greatest concern centres on the one in five men and women who are obese, because obesity is associated with elevated risk of chronic diseases and poor mental health. A woman with a body mass index (BMI) of 35 plus, which is medically classified as severe obesity, has a risk of developing type 2 diabetes up to 90 times compared to a normal weight woman (BMI 18.5–25). Severely obese men's risk of contracting this debilitating disease is only slightly less than that of women. Obesity is a risk factor for other conditions like coronary heart disease, cancer, stroke and arthritis (Cameron et al., 2003). Also, being overweight or obese increases the chance of having more than one of these conditions (Joint WHO/FAO Expert Consultation, 2003, p. 61).

The medical establishment is sufficiently alarmed and is in the process of shifting its attention from tobacco to obesity as the number one health risk in developed nations. According to the United States Centers for Disease Control and Prevention, the largest increase in deaths in that country in the last decade can be attributed to obesity and related conditions. While tobacco-related deaths are the number one cause of preventable death, obesity-related deaths are catching up fast. When the journal *Science* covered this story, they implied that, like tobacco use, those who are overweight have only themselves to blame. The opening lines went 'Sloth combined with bad diet may soon displace tobacco as the biggest cause of avoidable death in the United States ...' (Marshall, 2004, p. 804).

Globally, the situation is tending in the same direction, so that the major burden of disease will soon be attributed to obesity, even in developing societies. Already, the number of overweight and obese women in the world exceeds those who are underweight (Mendez et al., 2005), and developing countries are experiencing the double burden of poor nutrition: both under- and over-nutrition. This raises an unanswered question as to how public health agencies respond when households simultaneously contain members who are unhealthily overweight and underweight.

Australia's rates of obesity are approaching those of the United States and are among the highest in the developed world. Outside of the Middle East, the largest proportions of obese adults are mainly in English-speaking countries. In Britain, 'serious obesity' doubled between 1980 and 1991 (Prentice & Jebb, 1995). No one has yet explained this geopolitical trend, nor have they provided a satisfactory account for why the decade of the 1980s appears to have been the springboard for the rapid rise in global obesity. Based on material presented throughout this book, we speculate on that question in the competing authorities chapter.

Obesity over the lifecourse

A component of the rapid rise in obesity is its youthful onset with all the attendant co-morbidities. Twenty years ago, type 2 diabetes was unheard of among young people, but it is now appearing in children as young as ten years (Ebberling et al., 2002). The impact on the future burden of disease is likely to be significant because obese teenagers have a higher risk of becoming obese adults than normal-weight young people.

The preconditions for obesity are established early, possibly prior to conception. Maternal weight (or BMI) largely explains the association between birth weight and adult BMI in a British longitudinal study, which also suggested that maternal weight may be a more important risk factor for obesity in children than birth weight (Parsons et al. 1999). Although that possibility is yet to be confirmed, the three related points are better established:

- Birth weight is positively related to subsequent fatness (Parsons et al., 1999).
- Breastfeeding can prevent obesity in later life. Breastfed babies have a 30 per cent lower risk of obesity (Smith & Ingham, 2005).

- Childhood obesity is accompanied by risk of psychosocial problems: low self-esteem, social isolation, failure to engage with peers, schoolyard bullying and dissatisfaction with body image (French et al., 1995; Hill & Silver, 1995; Wake et al., 2002).

The prevalence of obesity among Australian children in 2001 was as high as 6 per cent, with one in every five children being either overweight or obese (Magarey et al., 2001). More alarming is the rate at which childhood obesity is increasing in Australia – over the course of the 20th century, the weight of Australian children rose on average by almost 1 kilogram per decade. This increase was most pronounced among the heaviest children (Olds & Harten, 2001). Between 1985 and 1997, there was a trebling of obesity among Australian children (Booth et al., 2003).

Other critical lifepoints (Gill, 1997) include early adulthood, in the years immediately after marriage, and around menopause. While it is natural to put on weight with age, rates of overweight and obesity are rising in all age groups. Obesity is most prevalent in the 45–64 year age group, but for the first time in history 70 year olds are not returning to normal weight status (Bennett, 2003). Later adulthood is when the weight-related complications for mobility are particularly marked, with osteoarthritis contributing to a spiral of social isolation and pain. The depression experienced by many older citizens could perhaps be exacerbated by physical symptoms associated with overweight.

Alternative conceptions of obesity

How one frames the issue of obesity influences both the research approach and the public policy response. And there is no shortage of competing theories to explain the causes, consequences and cures for obesity. Thus far we have provided the evidence-based portrayal of obesity as a health problem, but is the real problem the way the medical and public health field diagnose and discuss the issue of weight? By undertaking a decades-long content analysis of successive editions of a medical textbook, Chang and Christakis (2002) showed a marked shift in the medical field's attribution of responsibility for obesity. At the turn of the 20th century medical students were taught that obesity was something individuals brought on themselves through aberrant behaviour. Very gradually, this explanation has been displaced by theories that emphasise either genetic or environmental factors, both of which potentially free the individual from responsibility. Contemporary medical texts portray the obese as victims, but they offer competing remedies. If the social context is to blame, then the emphasis is one of environmental change; but if genetic disposition is to blame then biomedical remedies are required.

In a history of 20th-century American public health, Leichter (2003) notes that 80 years ago premature death was given collectivist explanations such as industrialisation, urbanisation and capitalism. With the consolidation of modernity, social aetiology was displaced by the idea of illness as 'a result of ignorance, laziness, immorality, or lack of willpower' (Leichter, 2003, p. 607). Other work supports the proposition that individualism is a hallmark of modernity (Eckersley, 2004), and the century ended with numerous examples of Australian governments ignoring collectivist explanations. Instead they have been exhorting citizens to adopt wiser lifestyles, and subsidising doctors to devise 'lifestyle scripts' for overweight patients. But this policy prescription only makes sense if 'people have the capacity and freedom to make wiser choices' once they leave the clinic (Leichter, 2003, p. 609).

The growth in obesity rates reveals a general failure to act effectively on medical and government advice. This failure is remarkable because of the daily presence of mass media images and stories that impugn the reputation of corpulent individuals as people who eat too much, exercise too little and lack self-control. The media sensationalise obesity through stories of the morbidly obese who cause enormous expense for public hospitals that must supersize their beds (Robinson & Creedy, 2004). At the same time, the fat person receives support from governments, industries and conservative commentators who champion an individual's freedom to choose to behave as they like (Pearson, 2003). In this sense, governments promote a contradictory message: lose weight but enjoy the market-based offerings that encourage weight gain.

The 'morally deficient' individual also receives support from another quarter. For members of the Size Acceptance Movement, as for Campos, the problem is not obesity but a culture-bound syndrome in societies characterised by a rejection of body fat and a worship of the skeletal. Sympathisers see body size as another basis for discrimination and they counter with a discourse on the rights of individuals of all sizes to be equally valued. For advocates of the overweight, the problem is lipophobia, or society's morbid fear of fat. Beginning in the United States in the late 1960s, the National Association to Advance Fat Acceptance (NAAFA) has provided a model for similar organisations in Australia and elsewhere. These movements have drawn support from public health campaigns to warn of the dangers of dieting (Sobal, 1999), including the establishment of an International No-Diet Day. The contemporary Size Acceptance Movement offers an individual-in-social context account of the situation, with members arguing that obesity is a normal response to an abnormal environment. This view of the evolution of the modern body lies at the heart of the increasingly popular ecological position in public health.

Ecologists argue that obesity is a consequence of consuming more and more energy at a time when energy expenditures have fallen dramatically. Obesity is thus best understood as the result of a mismatch between changes in living conditions and the needs and capacities of human biology (see McMichael, 2001). Our hunter-gatherer forebears led lives characterised by diets consisting of free-range animals, berries, fruits, nuts, tubers and leaves. These diets were not only high in protein, they were replete with unsaturated fats, some complex carbohydrates and less saturated fats, with no processed and refined carbohydrates (for example, sugar). Hunter-gatherers were also physically much more active. Following the domestication of plants and animals and a more regular and reliable food supply, a meal structure evolved that was highly specific to the immediate vicinity. Anthropologist Sidney Mintz (1994) has observed that in less than 150 years the aggressive promotion of two industrial products has eroded the agricultural meal structure. Previously marginal fats and processed sugars have displaced complex carbohydrates; and refined carbohydrates and animal-based proteins have become, in a brief period, the most prized of foods and a sign of progress the world over (Dixon, 2002).

In evolutionary terms, human metabolism is designed to make the most of energy and it has mechanisms that help to resist the loss of fat stores. The increase in appetite that occurs in response to a negative energy balance averts weight loss. However, mechanisms have never evolved to resist weight gain, perhaps because they were never required for species survival. This helps to explain why such an increase in obesity has been possible – weight gain can occur largely uninhibited by our genes, while the body resists weight loss. When there is a positive energy balance, that is when the amount of energy acquired is greater than the amount used, the excess energy is stored as fat. How much fat is stored is in part biologically or genetically determined. For example, biological correlates of age and sex play important roles. But genetics cannot explain the whole picture. It doesn't explain why there has been such a recent and rapid rise in obesity since 1980. And it doesn't explain why different social groups have different rates of obesity.

For a number of scientists, the post-World War II technological revolution that has ushered in cheaper food, car use and passive leisure, courtesy of the television and computer, is the pre-eminent cause of the recent rise in obesity (Prentice & Jebb, 1995; Reidpath et al., 2002; Reidpath et al., 2005). Other scientists place more emphasis on the process of urbanisation (Frumkin et al., 2004; Vandegrift & Yoked, 2004) and the attendant changes in consumption and lifestyle patterns brought about by easy access to industrial commodities and fewer rules governing their use. Irrespective of the causal emphasis, few dispute that human biology, while continuing to evolve, has been interacting with rapid changes in the social and physical environment, with repercussions for body shape and fat deposits.

In addressing the recent rise in obesity, Egger and Swinburn (1997) applied these ecological insights to establish an influential social ecological model of obesity. Their model describes how physical, political, social and cultural environments affect the behaviours of food consumption (for energy intake) and physical activity (for energy expenditure). Their term 'the obesogenic environment' describes a situation where the environment encourages energy intake and discourages energy expenditure (Swinburn et al., 1999). The concept has provoked a paradigm shift in how the multiple factors contributing toward obesity are understood. Still, too little attention is being paid to understanding which social actors and which social processes are contributing the most to making the environment obesogenic.

Thus, while we do not believe there is any single prime cause for the rapid change in average body size, we do believe that it is possible to identify and examine a set of inter-related social trends that are difficult for some groups to resist and easy for other groups to capitalise on. Within this highly charged context, we want to explain how individuals and groups are responding to the competing pressures to eat more and to eat less, to exercise more and to exercise less.

The seven 'original' and 'modern' sins of the individual

In the 13th century, Saint Thomas Aquinas spelt out seven major sins that afflicted 'mankind': pride, envy, avarice (greed), wrath, gluttony, sloth and lust. These sins became pivotal to religious and moral discourse, and they have crept unannounced into everyday and medical usage. Gluttony and sloth are invoked repeatedly by medical researchers to explain the 'obesity epidemic', even when they conclude that powerful environmental drivers, such as television and calorie-laden foods, underlie individual behaviours (Prentice & Jebb, 1995). Another of the sins, greed, is manifest in both the more morally tinged, mass media portrayals of the corpulent body as well as allegories of what makes 'the good life'. Thus, it is easy to invoke three of the seven deadly original sins on the path to obesity, and if pushed one could find a place for all of them. For example, an abundance of food is used by families, communities and individuals to symbolise wealth, to project pride and possibly to elicit envy. Similarly, a cornucopia is used artistically to foreground lust, and the spike in weight gain by newly marrieds might even be explained by the very original sin of lust. This leaves wrath, which makes its presence felt in the material on 'emotional eating' and eating disorders, when researchers note that individuals use food to compensate for all manner of emotional distress: they may binge-eat or spurn food to reflect self-loathing or cope with deep unhappiness.

Lying behind 'the sins' metaphor is an assumption that strong-willed individuals do not sin. And, the issue of self-control is never far from the surface in popular and academic accounts of obesity. In an economic model of self-control, Cutler and colleagues (2003) surmise that some people are more disposed to avail themselves of the abundance of ready-prepared foods, their version of the cornucopia. These 'impatient' people put off consideration of the health consequences of over-eating in favour of the immediate rewards from eating. Self-control also appears in explanations for why the more affluent are slimmer than other groups. Offer (2001, p. 91) suggests that where food satisfies the needs of lower socioeconomic groups by acting physiologically as an 'emotional tranquillizer', upper socioeconomic women in particular defer this form of gratification to remain slim, which they associate with greater sexual attractiveness and better job prospects. Slimmer men and women, by implication, practice greater self-control, and their lower body weight in turn operates to distinguish them as successful.

If overweight individuals renounced the seven sins would they be slimmer? We do not know of any study that has tested this hypothesis. However, at least in Britain, the public no longer see these particular sins as socially relevant. In a 2004 opinion poll conducted for the BBC television program 'Heaven and Earth', only 'greed' remained in the top seven sins. The other contemporary sins included: cruelty, adultery, bigotry, dishonesty, hypocrisy and selfishness (see www.mori.com/polls/2004/bbc-heaven.shtml). As the presenter of the program explained, people are now more concerned with actions that hurt others than with sins of indulgence per se. Perhaps discarding Aquinas's list of sins has opened the way to personal behaviours that lead to overweight.

While greed continues to be perceived as sinful, none of the six modern sins identified in the BBC poll discourages overconsumption or status competition via commodities. Thus, today's 'good life' could be virtuously replete with hedonistic pursuits, up to the point when greed kicks in. The British, and we assume other citizens of modern English-speaking countries, appear to be turning away from Weber's 'Protestant ethic' of hard work and self-denial, and embracing the pre-eminent expression of modern life, mass consumption (Eckersley, 2004), with mass consequences.

The seven 'modern' sins of the environment

As proponents of a social ecological perspective, we do not believe that obesity is a problem of sinful individuals, although part of the political solution must entail individuals acting to change their environments and their interactions with their environments if they wish to prevent weight gain. Instead, we place greater emphasis on the environmental determinants of obesity. Because of the ubiquitous debates concerning who is to blame for obesity, we propose that adopting the Seven Deadly Sins metaphor to focus attention on the social, cultural and physical environments may yield some traction in terms of public debate and policy response.

Our selection of what constitutes an environmental sin arises from a Delphi study conducted by a team at the National Centre for Epidemiology and Population Health (NCEPH) in 2003. In response to a question about 'the major social trends behind the rise in obesity in Australia in the last 50 years', 50 Australian experts in obesity and related fields agreed on the following top seven explanations for changes in physical activity and food consumption patterns:

- rising use of convenience and pre-prepared foods
- increasing 'busyness' and lack of time
- changing family dynamics
- sedentarisation of leisure activities
- escalating car reliance

- aggressive marketing of food
- changing knowledge, attitudes and practices in relation to physical activity (further details are reported in Banwell et al., 2005).

In reading the sociological, cultural and economic literatures relevant to these trends, we have recast the seven obesogenic trends nominated above as seven sins of modern environments. We argue that they exert influence over the social ecology and combine to generate significant detrimental impacts for health, including the rising prevalence of obesity. So exactly what are the seven deadly environmental sins?

THE COMMODIFIED ENVIRONMENT

Commodification refers to a transition away from the domestic production of foods and other household services to a consumer culture, based on reliance on commercially provided goods and services. The food service sector is not alone in contributing to the obesogenic environment. The leisure industry has shifted expectations about the correct way to spend 'free' time, with people allocating significant sums of money to 'taking a holiday' interstate or overseas, buying camping and sports equipment, and acquiring four-wheel drive cars (4WDs) to facilitate their recreation. Today's consumer culture encourages individualisation, as well as having a profound impact on how people think about what makes for a 'good life', leisure and the rewards of hard work.

THE HARRIED ENVIRONMENT

'Harriedness' incorporates the idea of time pressure plus being 'put-upon', or feeling oppressed and out of control. While harried people demand goods and services that help them to 'make time' and ease pressure, feeling harried is also partly a response to automation which allows people to fit more into a day. Indeed, how people define different forms of time (paid work, domestic work, leisure, free and discretionary time) influences their strategies to achieve work–family balance, including patterns of food consumption and physical activity. The complex web of social pressures to balance work–family commitments, with significant input from the market, is gradually shaping household food provisioning and activity patterns, with repercussions for weight gain.

THE PRESSURED PARENTING ENVIRONMENT

Since the 1950s, Dr Spock, Penelope Leach and others have preached the importance of putting the child at the centre of the household universe, proposing that children's development will be enriched if they are treated as autonomous human beings who are the best judge of their own needs. This is a marked departure from the parenting practices that preceded World War II. We outline how parenting practices and parental confidence have changed and how each child's individuality is being consolidated through commercial promotion of the 'junior consumer'. Data from France show that the autonomous child is not inevitable, and how that country's lower rates of obesity are a consequence of greater market regulation and a more rule-based family dynamic.

THE TECHNOLOGICAL ENVIRONMENT

Every social ill seems to have a technological solution, and this extends to 'solving' time famines, organising flexible work routines, providing childcare and taking exercise. Three technologies have been indispensable to everyday life in the last three decades: television, the microwave and the home computer. Television in particular plays a multifaceted role: as a marketing tool (especially to children), a form of childcare, and a harbinger of danger. We use the fixation on TV and other digital technologies as the cause of children's obesity to discuss whether children have become more sedentary in the last 50 years, and if so, whether these technologies are responsible.

THE CAR-RELIANT ENVIRONMENT

Cars are a further example of a modern technology used to remind people of the social and economic progress made over the 20th century. Like television, the car offers the chance for exercise-free transport and recreation and to consume heavily promoted commodities, especially fast food. The car has hitherto not attracted the same critical appraisal as television, but this may change as more research highlights the car's role in facilitating urban sprawl, which is associated with increasing rates of obesity in the United States and Australia. We describe the multiple ways in which car reliance shapes physical environments and public health, and how this particular practice is implicated in obesity.

THE MARKETED ENVIRONMENT

No Australian can escape the plethora of media exhortations to eat fast food, to buy a new car, to join commercial weight loss programs, and to consume convenience. But marketing, especially of foods, also takes more subtle approaches. We explore the tactics used by infant food producers to expand their market share at the expense of breastfeeding. This is a significant issue because infants who have been substantially breastfed are 30 per cent less likely to become obese in later life. We offer a detailed understanding of marketing, looking at how commercial infant food producers have taken advantage of opportunities created by 'scientific' childbirth and child-raising and by rising comparative economic 'costs' of breastfeeding to mothers.

THE ENVIRONMENT OF COMPETING AUTHORITIES

There has been a proliferation of groups dispensing conflicting advice about what constitutes a healthy diet and appropriate exercise. The traditional and moral authority of parents, adults, churches and professionals has been displaced by market-based authorities, including sports stars and other commercially sponsored experts. Many people have shifted from doing 'free' incidental exercise to paying for gym membership, personal trainers and exercise classes to help them undertake physical activity. They also seek advice from nutritionists, diet books and the Internet in a quest to find a slimming diet. As a result of the cacophony of voices competing to guide decisions, increasing numbers are either resigned to failure, are overtly repudiating the advice, or are so thoroughly confused as to become paralysed.

Book structure

Figure 1 provides a schematic model of the long causal chain that fosters obesity. The book's authors focus on the first three (upstream and midstream) determinants of obesity rather than on the individual responses to the social trends.

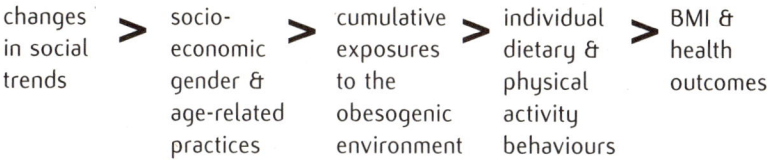

| changes in social trends | > | socio-economic gender & age-related practices | > | cumulative exposures to the obesogenic environment | > | individual dietary & physical activity behaviours | > | BMI & health outcomes |

FIGURE 1 A social ecological model of obesity

The chapters that follow describe the consequences of what it means to negotiate Australia's obesogenic environment. We show that a typical day in the life of the 'lucky' Australian is not the outcome of individual choice alone, but emerges from a complex web of environmental opportunities and constraints. For example, the Hinde chapter on car reliance describes how a privately owned means of transport is used to navigate sprawling suburbs to drop children at school, get to work, pick children up and drive them to after-school activities or to sit in front of television, while mothers rush into supermarkets for a heat-and-serve rotisserie chicken and fillings for tomorrow's school lunches. Such innocent activities can have profound health consequences for everyone.

Each of the seven environmental sins introduced above is described in a chapter. Denniss ('The commodified environment') shows that the ever-expanding economy lays foundations for the ever-expanding waistlines of the population, critiquing central assumptions of economic policy and theory. Broom and Strazdins ('The harried environment') argue that the modern phenomenon of time pressure, arising from the character of contemporary jobs and changing family life, undermines opportunities for the home-prepared meals and physical activity required for energy balance. This pattern relates directly to Banwell, Shipley and Strazdins's chapter ('The pressured parenting environment') because of the way time pressure contributes to the stressfulness of the responsibilities of being a parent, with consequences for children's weight. The decline of active leisure resulting from children and adolescents spending too much time with electronic gadgets – TV, computers and video games – supplies the focus for Dugdale and Dixon ('The technological environment'), who deconstruct the popular tendency for media and health experts alike to blame young people for unhealthy weight.

Technology has clearly contributed significantly to population weight increase, and the automobile is one of the most significant technologies in this regard. Hinde ('The car-reliant environment') shows how Australians have incorporated cars into their lives in many ways that affect their health. Smith's chapter on infant formula ('The marketed environment') argues that important seeds for rising obesity have been sown by breast-milk substitutes in infant feeding practices, a change driven by a close alignment between the commercial production and advertising of infant formulas and the beliefs and behaviours of health professionals who promoted the products, contributing to excess nutrition in the earliest months of life. This story is, in some senses, a specific example of a theme developed in the chapter by Dixon and Winter who outline the proliferation of competing authorities vying to instruct people in how to be healthy ('The environment of competing authorities'). In the penultimate chapter, Friel and Broom address how each of these seven deadly sins has contributed to different social groups having different body shapes, weight issues and states of health and wellbeing. It explains why rates of obesity have increased more for some groups – especially the poor, less educated, and Indigenous people – than others.

In the book's conclusion, the editors integrate the arguments, and suggest four actions to modify the physical and social environment, thereby enhancing the opportunities for individuals to exercise real choices about their body size.

Conclusion

It is possible that the public health focus on the 'obesogenic' environment shared by the contributors to this book may exacerbate the 'obesophobia' of contemporary culture. Although obesity is manifest in individuals, its root causes lie in the politics and priorities of the society, in such forms as food and transport systems, urban planning and design, the messages delivered by the media, and the organisation of work and leisure. The book approaches obesity as both a socioecological and political problem that must be addressed at the level of society.

With the aid of a broad sweep of the social sciences, we mount a case that to understand the social causes and consequences of the rapid rise in obesity, it is essential to focus on the changing social and physical environment. This book is devoted to halting further rises in obesity through influencing the nature of public discourse, policy calculations and public health responses to this complex issue.

SIN#1:
THE COMMODIFIED
ENVIRONMENT

How the economy feeds obesity

Richard Denniss

As lives in developed countries become increasingly removed from the natural world, the notion of consumption is being transformed. Whereas consumption once referred primarily to the intake of sustenance, it now refers to purchasing goods or services. Indeed shopping is sometimes even called 'food for the soul'. Citizens are increasingly referred to as 'customers' or 'consumers', even by government agencies who provide them with services (Torres et al., 2006). Such a transformation in the notion of what it means to consume is informative for the purposes of understanding the creation of an obesogenic society.

Societies were designed around the need to ensure adequate and stable food production, but that problem has long been solved in developed countries. Many of the best minds are no longer dedicated to the task of how to produce more; instead they are now concerned with how to sell more. This chapter argues that in an environment in which food is plentiful and technology substitutes for personal energy in many tasks, the imperative to maximise sales has dangerous implications for our physical, social and environmental health.

Economic historians have begun to analyse the impact of the

transformation from an agriculturally home-based provisioning system to the present reliance on commercially prepared 'convenience foods' (Chou et al., 2004; Cutler et al., 2003). Lower fixed costs of food preparation, combined with lengthening hours of paid work, have made the consumption of mass-produced foods more common.

This chapter discusses the link between growth in the economy and growth in waistlines and outlines the impact of 'consumer culture' on personal and public lives. First I provide an overview of the growth of the Australian economy with an emphasis on the widening scope of the economy as well as its increasing scale. That is, economic growth in Australia is not simply the result of producing more of the same goods and services that have always been produced. Instead, much of the growth has come from the rapid expansion of new sectors of the economy, particularly elements of the services sector. As more services, such as cooking and cleaning, that were once produced in the household sector are 'imported' into the home from the market, the economy is seen to expand and lifestyles are radically transformed. Home-cooked meals and takeaway meals differ not just in their supply of calories, but also in a wide range of accompanying attributes.

The second section introduces the impact of the assumption of 'non-satiety' inherent in contemporary economics (Hodgson, 2001). Put starkly, most economists assume explicitly that more is never enough, and that individual wellbeing is always enhanced when more is consumed compared to when less is consumed. While economists rely on their intuitive understanding of human nature as the basis for that assumption, their view conflicts with the concerns expressed by nutritionists and ecologists.

I go on to discuss the link between rising materialism, wasteful consumption expenditure and the need for more leisure time. I argue that leisure is personally and socially valuable but has become a 'commodity' relegated to the realm of a residual; that is, leisure time has come to be defined as the time left after people finish working, rather than as an end in itself. As leisure time has become scarcer, it has also become increasingly commodified. Whereas leisure once referred to the pursuit of an individual's passions, from stamp collecting to learning a musical instrument, it now refers more commonly to a holiday at the perfect beach resort.

The final section shows the impact of the overall trend towards consumerism on consumption patterns. It discusses how the process of commodifying social relationships has created a toxic personal and social environment. The impact of such trends on personal, family, community and national lives is discussed, as are the health implications.

Supersizing the Australian economy

The Australian economy grew by around $30 billion in 2005 (Australian Bureau of Statistics, 2006). That is, the value of all the goods and services bought and sold was around $30 billion greater than the value of the goods and services produced in 2004. The enormity of this increase in production is usually concealed through an emphasis on the percentage rate of growth in the size of the economy. The total value of all the goods and services bought and sold in Australia in 2005 was around $750 billion. When expressed in terms of such a large economy, the expansion in production can be referred to as a relatively modest 4 per cent rate of growth.

Australia is a rich country that becomes richer each year. But despite the fact that last year's growth affords the opportunity to solve an extra $30 billion dollars worth of problems, the vast majority of public and private discussions about spending focus on what the country cannot afford to do rather than what it can. If most economic debate is any indicator, Australians take for granted that solving the shortage of mobile phones among 16 year olds is a national priority while paying lip service to the notion that more should be done to improve Indigenous health outcomes (if only the money were available).

While the capacity to produce more has risen steadily in recent decades, demand for goods and services has risen even faster. In a marketing culture like this one, images of what people do not have are everywhere, while reminders of good fortune are few and far between. Older generations may hold on to quaint notions about the virtue of saving for the future, spending wisely and avoiding waste, but younger generations have formed their worldview in a social environment dominated by recreational shopping, ease of access to credit cards and a boom in advertising targeted directly at children. This contrast should not be used as a basis to disparage younger generations as selfish or materialistic. It was, after all, their parents' generations who – without appreciating the consequences – created the environment of commercial consumption.

While the size of the economy and its rate of growth are much discussed in policy and business circles, its scope should be of most interest to social scientists. Economic growth does not result only from expansion in particular forms of production; it can also occur when new forms of production are developed or when old forms of production once considered outside the realm of 'the economy' are incorporated into the definition of the market.

New forms of production emerge continuously, sometimes in response to technological change, sometimes in response to changes in fashion. Two decades ago there was no commercial Internet; now activity on the Internet contributes billions of dollars to the national economy (DCITA, 2005). Similarly, five years ago few school age boys would have spent $100 on having their hair cut and coloured. Today, such demand adds millions of dollars to measured economic growth.

An important issue that is rarely debated in Australia is the extent to which markets respond to consumer demands, and how far consumers respond to the advertising of new products. Did consumers demand larger portion sizes at restaurants, or did restaurants offer larger portions as an effective way to market themselves as providing 'good value for money'? In an environment where expenditure on marketing continues to grow rapidly, and the advertising industry is forecast to grow by 9.6 per cent in 2006 to $10.3 billion (Lee, 2005), the absence of such a debate impedes the development of both good public understanding and good public policy.

However, the focus of this chapter is not on the impact of marketing new products (see chapters by Smith and by Dixon and Winter), but rather on the way old forms of production have become marketised. The benefits of adolescent expenditure on hair colouring are rightly debatable, but there is no doubt about the flaws in a system of national accounts that ignores the value of unpaid work done within the home and counts the value of those same activities when an external party is paid to perform them.

When people grow fruit in their back yard and eat it, this production and consumption is considered to be of no value by those responsible for measuring gross domestic product (GDP). But when someone drives to the shop to purchase fruit, even if they throw it away rather than eat it, they will have contributed to the economy. As families spend less time preparing their own meals and cleaning their own houses, these services that were once considered by economists to be, quite literally, worthless are now redefined as an important source of economic growth.

The marketisation of household production exaggerates the rate of economic growth, and in turn overstates the rate of 'progress'. A portion of what is measured as increased production in Australia is simply a measurement error caused by the policy choice to attach zero value to non-market production within the home yet include the full price paid when external labour is hired to perform those same tasks. An old joke among economists is that when a man marries his housekeeper the economy shrinks.

Thus, economic accounting is often a poor proxy for the welfare of the population. But the problems are not confined to measurement alone. The marketisation of what was once considered to be 'household work' has a fundamental impact on the creation of knowledge and on the construction of social relationships. Most children have no idea how much sugar and fat are required to bake a cake. Many adults are similarly unaware, either because they too have never made a cake, or because it has been so long that they have forgotten.

Britain's 'Naked Chef' Jamie Oliver recently provoked outrage when he was shown slaughtering a lamb in a TV cooking program. Oliver reasoned that a man who had cooked over 2000 sheep in his career should at least have the courage to kill one. This argument was not well received by numerous viewers who found his behaviour 'barbaric'. This reaction illustrates how remote many modern urban people have become from the processes required to deliver products – including meat – to the market and the dinner table, and how the market limits public knowledge of what are sometimes unpalatable or otherwise unpleasant aspects of these hidden processes.

Household production is intimate, personal and negotiated. Market production is based on the idea that the division of labour is the most efficient form of production. Consequently, market production is diffuse, impersonal and distant. This is not to say that the conduct and division of household work is always rewarding and fair, or that market production is inherently undesirable and unfair. Housework is often unjustly allocated, and there are market relationships in which friendship and trust develop. Nevertheless, the increasing scope of market production and the declining amount of time allocated to household production are likely to have significant effects on individuals, households and the community more generally. As Barbara Pocock puts it:

> Mutual non-monetary exchanges have embedded within them – indeed create – personal and community relationships. These obligations are the stuff of community and generalised reciprocity. They create trust and long term witnesses to one's life. (Pocock, 2003)

More is never enough

The Australian economy has grown rapidly and, by historic standards, steadily for the last decade (Australian Bureau of Statistics, 2006). But the fact that Australians are, by world standards, rich and getting richer, has not been able to shift the focus to other personal or social problems. In fact, for economists at least, it is inconceivable that people could ever have 'enough'.

Mainstream economics is based on a number of axioms, one of the least widely understood of which is euphemistically referred to as 'non-satiety'. The assumption of non-satiety literally implies that 'rational economic agents' can never be satisfied. Owning one car is inherently less desirable than owning two. Twenty pairs of shoes must be preferable to fifteen pairs. And ominously, when faced with the choice of eating 2 kilograms of chocolate or 3, economic theory asserts that the latter is axiomatically superior.

The assumption of non-satiety holds at both the microeconomic level (the individual) and at the macroeconomic level (the national economy). Both individuals and the nation are always assumed to be better off if they have more rather than less.

As an axiom, the belief in non-satiety need not be empirically verified in order for most economists to place implicit faith in its descriptive power. Given the economic problems of scarcity that have confronted humanity throughout most of history, it is perhaps understandable why such an assumption has remained unchallenged. A society like Australia cannot, however, continue to conceal the conflict between the assumption of non-satiety and the assumption that a balanced diet is an essential precondition for good personal and public health outcomes. Similarly, there is a conflict between the desire for ever greater levels of production and environmental sustainability, including an urban environment characterised by peace, quiet, fresh air, and opportunities for recreational physical activity and active transport.

The idea that more is better permeates both private behaviour and public policy. The 'supersize me' marketing strategy has been subject to sustained attack in recent years, but despite the current critique of such marketing practices, they still persist and reveal much about Western consumer behaviour.

When faced with two choices, an adequate quantity for a reasonable price or an enormous quantity for slightly more, many people will choose the latter, believing it to represent 'better value'. Coulter and Coulter (2005) conducted experiments on test subjects and concluded that serving size not only affected perception of value, but that consumers were not consciously aware of this relationship. This result was confirmed by Burger King in an in-house analysis of their upsizing strategy. They found that:

> 'Bundled meals offer the greatest cost savings to consumers while also offering a greater profit margin for restaurants,' said Dana Frydman, senior director, product marketing for Burger King Corporation. 'Historically, fries and beverages have a greater penny profit margin than sandwich entrees,' she said ...

> With the 'Make It A Meal' promotion, Burger King® customers have the option of trading-up to the Large Value Meal which features a New large fry and large soft drink for 40¢ more or

the King Value Meal which includes a NEW 'bigger' King size fry plus a NEW King size soft drink for 80¢ more ...

Research shows that consumers rate Value Meals as the second most important reason – behind restaurant location – for selecting a quick-service restaurant and consumers who purchase value meals generally seize the opportunity to upsize. (QSR, 2006)

Despite consumers having purchased more than they originally intended or would have objectively determined they needed, the sense of value stems from what they have gained from the supplier rather than the relationship between their 'needs' and the quantity purchased. Movie theatres employ this strategy at its most extreme, with popcorn and soft drink containers growing exponentially, and such strategies are now employed broadly. Petrol stations typically offer two chocolate bars for slightly more than the price of one, DVD rental stores offer three movies for slightly more than the price of one, and exercise studios offer 12 months membership for slightly more than the price of three months. It seems that the search for a 'bargain' can lead to consuming more than one might otherwise have planned.

At the macroeconomic level, a tendency to over-consume is generally seen as 'good for the economy' rather than bad for health or for the natural environment. Attempts to control advertising of soft drinks to children typically attract derision often backed up with evidence about the importance of the food industry to the economy. And in a political environment that assumes the economy can never be big enough, the assertion that something will reduce the size of the economy dominates all other arguments.

Many commentators acknowledge that rising obesity rates are closely linked to the over-riding priority given to economic growth, whose pursuit induces and demands ever-increasing private consumption. This nexus can be seen in the many ways obesity itself contributes to national economies. For example, the United States produces 140 per cent of its food requirements, generating powerful incentives to high levels of consumption both at home and abroad. Enormous amounts are spent on advertising to encourage excessive food consumption (McDonald's spends

US$1 billion on advertising each year). Tens of millions are spent on diet programs, pills and liposuction (Campos, 2004). There are considerable healthcare costs associated with obesity.

In a bizarre twist, obesity is a drain on societal resources (mainly as a result of the associated healthcare costs and the loss of working age people from the workforce) even as it fuels economic activity. As with tobacco-related taxes, governments stand to gain from company taxes paid as a result of profits on food, advertising, dieting and medical intervention (Chopra & Darnton-Hill, 2004).

In any event the solution to the growing problem of obesity is likely to involve much more than simply restricting advertising. Public drinking fountains may need to replace soft drink vending machines once again in schools, train stations and workplaces. Food labelling may have to declare energy content in terms of how many 'standard meals' a product contains, just as bottles of alcohol now do for 'standard drinks'. And exercise may have to be designed into daily life, in the form of carless city centres and bike paths with priority over car lanes (Cevero & Duncan, 2003; Frumkin et al., 2004).

An understanding of the assumption of non-satiety in orthodox economics helps explain how radical and (in the short term at least) how unlikely such proposals are to attract political support when economic perspectives dominate. The problem is that solutions like those above not only face opposition from individual industries: they go to the heart of the modern socioeconomic system. Policy solutions that encourage people to spend less money would result in slower economic growth, if only in a particular industry. Such solutions, therefore, are likely to be politically costly.

Your money or your life?

Contradictions between a healthy economy and a healthy population are evident not only in political decisions, but also in personal decision-making (as susceptibility to the super size 'bargains' illustrates). Such thinking seems to structure people's choices about time as well as about the products themselves.

When people in full-time work were asked whether they would prefer to have a 4 per cent pay rise or an additional two weeks paid annual leave, 51 per cent of those surveyed said they would prefer to have the additional paid leave. That is, when individuals are confronted with a specific choice between time and money, more than half of full-time employees opt for more time (Denniss, 2003). Yet surprisingly, less than 1 per cent of employees actually act on such preferences.

There are few Australians who believe that money is more important to their happiness than their health or their families. The problem is that most people do not make decisions about money, family and health in a co-ordinated way. People who take a promotion because they 'need' more money are unlikely to have decided that they 'need' to spend less time with their family or less time taking care of their health. Yet that can be the consequence.

Why do so few people actually purchase additional leave even when it is available? While it is possible that actions speak louder than words (and that people don't really value time over money), there is a wide range of evidence that individuals experience both personal and structural barriers to pursuing additional leave. Many workers already struggle to access the four weeks leave to which they are entitled. The major reasons for failing to take leave are either that they were too busy at work or that their boss would not give them time off that suited their needs (Denniss, 2003). Further, many workers believe, rightly or wrongly, that seeking additional leave signals a lack of commitment to either the organisation or to one's work colleagues, and some of their managers may subscribe to the same view.

For over 20 years Australian politics has been dominated by the deregulation of the labour market and the drive to make it more 'flexible'. Yet, despite the rhetoric of flexibility and individual choice that has dominated these public debates, people who express a choice for more leisure time are either stigmatised as lazy or prevented from achieving their preferences either by recalcitrant managers or by structures designed to ensure that individual choices operate within a constrained set of options.

As society gets richer, people can either buy more things or have more leisure time. Given the putative link between long work hours, poor diet and physical health (see the chapter by Broom and Strazdins), a shift in preferences away from buying 'stuff' and towards buying time is likely to yield significant health improvements. Such a shift is also likely to at least slow the rate of environmental damage.

It is important to note that 'leisure' (what the Australian Bureau of Statistics [ABS] calls 'free time') does not imply holiday travel. Like most human activities, leisure time has become highly commodified in recent decades, with the result that for many people talk of increased leisure time elicits images of more international travel, 4WDs towing caravans, trail bikes and jet skis.

The primary meaning of leisure was once 'the pursuit of one's passions'. For many it has now become 'the pursuit of time on the couch'. The objective of this chapter is to begin a debate around the need for not just an increase in leisure time but a redefinition of leisure time. For example, does retail shopping on public holidays reflect a passion for this form of leisure or does it represent the fact that other forms of passing time and being active have not been promoted as satisfying and rewarding socially and economically?

To improve population and environmental health, the pursuit of increased leisure time should be seen as a legitimate and desirable choice. The case for labour market deregulation by economic rationalists was that individuals are best placed to make their own decisions about what is best for them. The rhetorical line of conservative politicians in Australia is that investing more heavily in family relationships is essential in order to preserve the 'Australian way of life'. The church has always said that money does not buy happiness and that people need to search for deeper meaning in their lives. Yet people who seek to work less in order to improve their lives and the lives of their families are likely be met with complaints from conservatives and economic rationalists that their behaviour is selfish and irresponsible.

Leisure time is an important component of physical and emotional health. It is also an essential ingredient in the construction and maintenance of a sense of community. People are bombarded with messages about the need for new, bigger and better material things. Individuals form expectations and desires in part through their observation of, and interaction with, other individuals. The role of leisure in a 'successful' life seems to have been relegated to the realm of retirement. Having worked hard all one's life, one can then relax and enjoy the fruits of that labour. Unfortunately, even this message is propagated by the retirement savings industry that seeks to encourage people to save up ever larger 'nest eggs' to fund their retirement consumption and leisure activities. In fact, good health and good relationships are as essential to an enjoyable retirement as a good bank balance.

Consuming passions

Even though Australians are richer, they are working longer than ever before (Denniss 2003). At the same time concern about the need for more time with families has emerged as a significant social issue (Pocock, 2003). This conflict could be explained by oppressive employers imposing greater demands on their employees, but such oppression, if it exists, is difficult to discuss publicly given the widespread use of the term 'flexibility' in reference to the modern Australian labour market. Either desires for more time at work and more time at home are contradictory, or the language for discussing such desires is. For most people, the answer is probably a combination of both.

A similar contradiction emerges when considering the stated desire of Australians to help reduce their environmental impact alongside the individual consumption choices and collective political choices that most Australians make. Most Australians express strong support for the need to reduce greenhouse gas emissions (Greenpeace, 2002), but the trend towards larger cars and houses has continued apace.

Finally, most Australians say that they want to live a healthier lifestyle and do more exercise yet participation in physical activity continues to decline and levels of obesity continue to rise (Australian Institute of Health and Welfare [AIHW] 2004). Either people are in denial about their real preferences, or socioeconomic forces are such that individual preferences are no match for social pressures.

The individual is held in high esteem in a consumer culture. In fact, the capacity of market economies to provide individuals with 'choice' is usually perceived to be the strongest benefit associated with market capitalism (see for example Hayek, 1972; Herzlinger, 2002). Economists insist that individuals are expressing their free will to make the best choices. This rhetoric is used frequently to discredit other forms of social organisation, particularly the direct provision of services by 'nanny state' governments or the imposition of 'red tape' regulation that restricts the nature of choices offered to consumers.

But while personal choice can be a good thing, there are many instances in which choice is widely perceived to be undesirable. Most consumers, for example, express reluctance, if not hostility at the thought of having to spend time 'choosing' their electricity supplier or the 'most suitable' credit card for them. Even strong advocates of neoliberalism and the benefits of choice often find themselves arguing against the provision of individual choice when it comes to the decision to take illicit drugs or seek the termination of a pregnancy.

Thus, it is meaningless to argue about whether the abstract notion of choice is desirable or not. In order to assess the desirability of choice it is necessary to consider the environment in which choices are to be made. Australians say they would like to work less, spend more time with their families, do more exercise and help to protect the environment. Unfortunately, evidence suggests they are working longer hours, spending less time with their families, doing less exercise and doing more harm to the environment (Australian Institute of Health and Welfare (AIHW), 2005; Denniss, 2003; Hamilton, 2003).

Of course it is possible to dismiss the stated concerns of individuals and focus on their behaviour. Such an approach is referred to by economists as a focus on 'revealed preferences', the term being used to distinguish between what people say they want and what they really want. But an alternative approach is to assume that when discovered contradictions between stated desires and behaviour are substantial, then we need to consider the context in which choices are being made. For example, the 'need' for children to have a mobile phone is as dependent on the decisions made by other children to have a phone as it is on the features and benefits of a mobile phone. Similarly, individual decisions to buy large 4WD vehicles are likely to be as influenced by other people's decisions to buy such vehicles as they are by the 'inherent' desire to own one.

Another axiom relied on by economists is that of 'independence'. That is, economists explicitly assume that the preferences and desires of individuals are independent of each other. There is no room in the standard economic analysis for any form of 'interdependence' of desires; that is, there is no room in the model for peer pressure, fads, fashion or community norms.

A decision to cook more meals at home has implications for an individual's negotiations about hours of work with their employer. The desire to spend more time in the kitchen will be hard to achieve for a person who decides to swap their 4WD for public transport. Cars may be polluting and expensive, but for most people they deliver the shortest commuting times, and simplify complicated lives (see Hinde chapter). Similarly, the desire to reduce car use and help reduce greenhouse gasses has implications for the amount of time a person can spend participating in community activities or visiting relatives and friends.

Modern lives are highly interdependent. Work and spending decisions are deeply related to transport decisions. Decisions about personal relationships have an enormous impact on housing. Changing one element of one's life can be difficult as it is likely to have substantial effects on other areas of life. Consumerism exacerbates this problem. Consumerism is biased towards selling solutions rather than solving problems at their source, and the more time pressured and emotionally stressed people become the more likely they are to settle for a soothing short-term balm rather than implement a more difficult long-term solution.

Overworked and tired people seek the expensive solace of weekend trips away or visits to a day spa. The short-term relief is apparent, but the impact on the credit card makes the idea of working shorter hours and earning less money seem impossible. Tired and busy people are more likely to consume multi-vitamin pills and energising extracts added to their $5 fruit juices than to rethink their decision to buy a house where walking or cycling to work was impossible. Once again, the environment in which decisions are made is important. For example, poor urban design encourages short-term solutions, regardless of their health consequences (Cevero & Duncan, 2003).

Conclusion

The solutions to the emerging personal and social problems associated with overwork, under-exercising, overeating and under-investing in relationships are unlikely to be offered in the form of a consumer product or self-help service. But the provision of these kinds of 'choices' focuses attention on the role of the individual, and their personal capacity to cope, rather than on the structural causes of those same problems. Individuals must accept responsibility for making good decisions, but societies must also take responsibility for ensuring that individuals can make healthy choices in a healthy environment. However, to solve these problems at the social level requires overcoming one important obstacle: the process of solving problems is not nearly as profitable as producing goods for temporary, symptomatic mitigation. Consumerism will often provide a temporary solution to life's problems, but it rarely provides an answer, and it is a key contributor to rising obesity in a population.

SIN#2:
THE HARRIED
ENVIRONMENT

Is time pressure making us fat?

Dorothy H Broom and Lyndall Strazdins

If sloth is a sin, is being busy the virtue to counteract it? And is it busyness (not sloth) that is making us fat? Western societies have a strong cultural imperative toward being busy. Weber's famous treatise *The Protestant Ethic and the Spirit of Capitalism* outlines how a broad cultural trend toward valuing diligence was internalised by a growing portion of the population and in turn fostered the growth of a capitalist political economy. Once in place, this symbiotic relationship became self-perpetuating. The recent trend toward materialism is, according to some analyses, a logical consequence of the unrivalled ascendancy of capitalism in the late 20th century. While the earlier emphasis on 'salvation by works' may have receded, people in Anglo and European societies continue to be encouraged to become diligent, hard working and acquisitive. The term 'aspirational' signals the cultural and political emphasis placed on such values.

Contemporary life is full of references to speed, time pressure and rushing. During the 1950s and 1960s, the introduction of computers and automated production, along with the long-term decline in hours at work, prompted forecasts of a coming 'leisure society'. The problem would be how to spend the excess of free time people would have by the end of the century. Paradoxically, in the new millennium time poverty, time pressure and overwork are the palpable social issues, rather than too much free time. People report having too much to do, and both popular (Gleick, 1999) and academic (Schor, 1992) books debate the issue. So a discourse was readily available to the 50 Australian experts who nominated 'time pressure' when they were asked to propose the social trends that have contributed most to the rise in obesity over the last half century (see this book's introduction). Indeed, one in five experts ranked time pressure as the single most important cause (Banwell et al., 2005).

But how could time pressure influence people's weight? Because healthy weight requires a balance between energy consumption and expenditure, perhaps when people are busy, it is hard to engage in the behaviours necessary for energy balance and they will be liable to gain weight. But are Australians really being time pressured into getting fat?

The question can be addressed in three ways. First, time pressure could increase weight because it limits exercise time, increases intake of energy-dense foods (which are quick to acquire and eat) and limits the time available to prepare less energy-dense alternatives. This is a straightforward argument: doing things to maintain healthy weight takes time, and so time pressure will result in unhealthy weight. As one participant in the Delphi exercise observed, people now '... have to prioritise to fit activity into the day'. And eating fast food on the run was another theme mentioned frequently in that study.

A second possibility (a refinement of the first) is that time pressure only increases the risk for obesity for some people, under certain conditions, and at certain points in history. Time pressure is one of several converging trends, and on its own might be only loosely related to weight. But taken in combination with other trends – sedentary jobs, abundant high energy food, sedentary transport – time pressure becomes pivotal. By this view, having lots to do is not a recent invention. Two hundred years ago people were busy too, but their jobs and their transport involved high energy expenditures. Now, most jobs and transport are sedentary, and high energy food is abundant. Making time for physical activity must be squeezed into schedules already filled with jobs, family care, transport, and so adds a time cost – and this is why time pressure becomes the key.

Finally, time pressure might simply be another modern malaise, unrelated to obesity, that happens to be occurring at the same time, and indeed may not even be a real phenomenon. Thus when the experts discussed the links in more detail, the mechanisms they mentioned were quite subtle and sometimes contradictory. Several proposed that increased busyness was a perception rather than a reality of modern life. Others described a variety of social and economic changes that exert pressure on the allocation of people's time, but these appeared to have little if anything to do with weight gain. For example, one expert noted that going out for fast food 'takes as long as making a salad sandwich,' but that people may not perceive it that way, especially if they have little experience in basic food preparation.

The relationships between time pressure and obesity may in fact encompass all the above, with contradictory and subtle combinations. For example, time pressure may prompt people to both skip meals and to rely on energy-dense fast food. It may discourage the use of active transport, but also be the result of exercising. Some people may be busy in part because they have regular sessions with a personal trainer. Deadlines at work may make people feel they are too busy to eat (reducing energy input), so they stay at their desk instead of going out of the office (reducing energy output).

In this chapter we review these possibilities. We consider if time pressure is increasing, and if so, why. Then we turn to the evidence linking time pressures to health behaviours that underpin obesity, particularly exercise and physical activity, and the consumption of high energy food. Finally, we briefly consider whether these links are universal, or might mainly apply to some people, at certain points of the lifecourse, facing particular combinations of demands and pressures. (Some of these possibilities are investigated in more depth in the chapter by Banwell and colleagues.)

Are Australians becoming busier?

Some writers attribute rising time pressure to urbanisation and industrialisation generally. It is suggested that factories and cities, by their nature, make life busier than it is on farms, in villages or in small towns. The pre-industrial household was a site of irregular, seasonal and task-oriented labour; industrialisation standardised time and thus generated the distinction between 'work' and 'life' (Thompson, 1967). However, the advent of scientific management during the late 19th and early 20th centuries receives particular emphasis. With its focus on efficiency and punctuality as mechanisms to organise and control work (domestic and paid) (Davison, 1993), it is thought to have laid the industrial and psychological foundations for today's 'epidemic' of time stress. The commodification of time itself ('time is money') may contribute to the contemporary sense of time pressure (Gross, 1984).

There seems little doubt that people *feel busier* now than they did 50 years ago. Investigating this is, however, complicated by the possibility that being busy has become a signifier of status and hence something people may be motivated to claim whether they feel busy or not (Gershuny, 2005). Nevertheless, an abundant literature testifies to the widespread psychological experience of having too much to do in the time available (Hochschild, 1997; Schor, 1992), and those who feel harried are not always the elite. A survey by Statistics Canada found that 'one third of employed mothers are "extremely time stressed" and more than 70 per cent feel rushed on a daily basis' (Colman, 1999). Feeling rushed is both widespread and became more common during the last quarter of the 20th century, in the United States at least (Robinson & Godbey, 1999; Sayer, 2005; Sayer & Mattingly, forthcoming). Several technical innovations contribute directly to rising time consciousness: computers displaying the time, wristwatches with alarms, telephones that time calls, fitness equipment that monitors time, maps that signal distance in travel time as well as (or instead of) distance, packaged foods and recipes emphasising speed of preparation (Davison, 1993). By some accounts, it is this subjective experience of time pressure that counts (Mann & Tan, 1993). However, other commentators prefer what they regard as more 'objective' measures.

Hours in the day:
The loss of discretionary time

One measure of time pressure is the daily allocation of hours, but even that hardly tells a simple story. Technological change and union campaigns produced the 20th century's long decline in paid work hours (Nyland, 1986). Depending on how it is measured, some observers insist that the trend towards shorter working hours continues, at least in some nations (JP Robinson & Godbey, 2005; Wooden, 2001), although by some accounts, the United States and Australia may be exceptions to the pattern in most developed economies (International Labor Organization, 1999). In the latter part of the century in Australia, hours for full-time workers began to increase once again as part of a generalised move away from the 'standard working week' (Australian Bureau of Statistics, 2003; Wooden, 2001) and towards increased diversity in working patterns: more part-time workers (who reduce total average working hours) alongside an increasing proportion of full-time employees who work more than 40 or even 50 hours per week. This growing divide has complex implications for the time people have available because it is imperfectly related to differences in pay. People working long hours are often also well paid and hence in a position to purchase goods and services (nannies, high-quality catered food, domestic help, chauffeurs) that partly compensate for their time on the job. By contrast, employees with fewer paid work hours may have more unpaid time available, yet much of that apparently 'free' time must be allocated to performing the functions that better paid workers can pay someone else to do (childcare, shopping, cleaning, and so on). A model developed by Goodin and colleagues, and applied to Australian time use survey data, shows (not surprisingly) that lone parents are the most liable to be time poor (Goodin et al., 2002).

The academic debate over whether time pressure has 'really' risen revolves partly around questions of measurement, and partly around the interpretation of measures. Underlying the debate are numerous methodological, conceptual and political or values commitments (not always explicitly stated). We do not resolve the debate, but present the most prominent questions and explore how they might be implicated in health-related behaviour and particularly in weight.

Fragmentation, multitasking, colonisation and time management

Both the *speed* of activity and the *density* of scheduling are correlated with busyness (Levine, 2005). In addition to the feeling of being busy, and the hours spent doing paid and unpaid work, another element of time pressure is the *fragmentation* of waking hours into multiple and often simultaneous activities (Floro & Miles, 2001). Parents (especially mothers, who are usually responsible for childcare and domestic work) are particularly likely to resort to *multitasking* to cope with the numerous different tasks they must perform (Bittman & Wajcman, 2000). Eating or putting on make-up while driving, and combining housework and childcare are familiar examples.

Closely related is a phenomenon known as the *colonisation* of time – that is, the gradual erosion of the boundary between work and home or leisure – and there is evidence that children resent it when parents bring work home (Pocock & Clarke, 2004). Of course the home has always been a site of unpaid labour for women (Broom, 1986), but increasingly paid work now also comes home. Technological change and the globalisation of business both contribute significantly to this process. The availability of the fax machine, mobile phone, laptop and Internet/telecommuting have created circumstances in which workers are now accessible 24/7, and may indeed be working at any hour of any day, sometimes with co-workers who are thousands of kilometres and many time zones distant. Australian time-use research suggests that women's 'free' time is particularly vulnerable to being combined with (or colonised by) household work and childcare (Bittman & Wajcman, 2000), and this pattern is also evident in United States research (Mattingly & Bianchi, 2003).

The combination of density, fragmentation, multitasking and colonisation generates a complex new chore for many people, namely the need to *manage* and co-ordinate competing priorities and the multiple demands of family members and colleagues. In families, this management responsibility generally falls to mothers who must negotiate the various personal and transport trajectories generated by the diverse commitments of their family members. In professional settings, a personal assistant performs this function for senior managers. Dual-earner households must often resort to an emphasis on 'efficiency' in their daily life in order to deal with time pressure (Brown & Warner-Smith, 2005).

Because work, social and even familial networks tend to be more widely dispersed geographically than they once were, it appears that a new (or at least amplified) task has come onto the modern social agenda: fostering network connections. Increasingly, people telecommute or work with colleagues in distant locations. Patterns of marital separation and blended families generate more complex webs of 'family fragments' that require negotiation and management. Overall, 'more "work" has to be put into nurturing such networks since there is less casual interaction; when people do meet face-to-face this often involves travel across substantially longer distances' (Cass et al., 2005).

Social and economic trends underlying time pressure

Some writers have argued that for most people, the distressing feeling of being 'time poor' is largely self-inflicted, a product of rising social and material expectations (Greenfeld, 2005) rather than being imposed by circumstances beyond people's control, and indeed some of the experts in the Delphi exercise articulated this view. According to this logic, people are free to change the disposition of their time if they are unhappy with their level of time pressure, and there is limited empirical evidence that some Australians are doing just that (Hamilton & Mail, 2003). A national survey found that 23 per cent of people in the prime working ages (30–59) had made a *voluntary* long-term change (apart from planned retirement) that resulted in a lower income and, one assumes, reduced time pressure. Improved 'balance' and more time for family were frequently mentioned as reasons for this downshifting. If this trend is confirmed, it suggests that at least some people can make more time for family and other non-work commitments if they are able and willing to forfeit some income.

However, it is important not to romanticise this process since some forms of downshifting can entail substantial sacrifice. For example, moving from full-time to part-time employment may involve underemployment (taking a job for which the worker is overqualified) (Darton & Hurrell, 2005), and could leave people with inadequate retirement income later. While it appears that people may be able to diminish busyness by reducing their level of material consumption (and perhaps job satisfaction), countervailing trends indicate that some of the sense of time pressure is not so readily relinquished, or not by everyone anyway (Ehrenreich, 2001). In addition to the lone mothers identified by Goodin and colleagues, some employees may be required by their employers to work long (and sometimes unsociable) hours as a condition of getting or keeping a job. When this happens, people may be under a kind of invisible time pressure where they are not compelled by their formal work contract to be on the job for excessive hours, but the informal workplace culture imposes a different set of demands. Several of the retail and public service managers we have interviewed for a study of working conditions and family health have observed that arriving early, staying late and being available on call 24/7 are effectively non-negotiable (but tacit) requirements for promotion to management positions. Declining adequacy and entitlement to welfare-state support may act synergistically to make it riskier to refuse demands to work long hours, or to opt for downshifting, because people feel anxious about providing for their families. Thus, while people may enjoy a kind of theoretical freedom to reduce their level of time pressure, in practical terms, that freedom may be much more limited than it seems.

Some limitations may operate simultaneously within and outside the scope of any individual or household's control. Unilaterally overthrowing personal and cultural values and norms is exceptionally rare because it is exceedingly difficult, requiring a large measure of critical self- and social-awareness, and perhaps – paradoxically in this instance – a considerable amount of free time to reflect on the consequences of acceding to prevailing norms and patterns.

Health effects of time pressure

In light of the evidence for increasing time pressure, we turn now to the question of how such pressure might be related to health generally and to unhealthy weight in particular. Fully comparative data are not available, but some evidence indicates that excessive weight occurs more often among people who are experiencing time pressured circumstances. For example, parents (especially mothers) with young children both sleep less and devote less time to leisure activities than other adults (Craig & Bittman, 2005). Parents (especially mothers) in dual-earner households (Brown & Warner-Smith, 2005) and lone mothers are particularly likely to have to make such trade-offs, and insufficient leisure is likely to reduce levels of physical activity.

People in paid work are under more time pressure than other adults, and there are suggestions that obesity is more prevalent among workers (Medibank Private, 2005). This Australian survey also reported that workers had lower prevalence of adequate physical activity, and of fruit and vegetable consumption.

Earlier, we described the trend towards longer work hours. When work is sedentary, this translates into increased exposure to a key risk factor for obesity and physical inactivity. People whose jobs are literally sedentary (with long sitting times) have poor long-term subsequent levels of physical functioning (Leino-Arjas et al., 2004) and higher prevalence of excess weight (Mummery et al., 2005; Proper et al., 2006) than people whose jobs involve less sitting. Furthermore, the association predicts an elevated risk of death from ischaemic heart disease (Salonen et al., 1988). Compared to physical activity, there is as yet less evidence linking time pressure specifically to the consumption of energy-dense food, even though the association between being rushed and using fast food makes sense intuitively, and a tendency to eat energy-dense foods when under stress has been empirically documented (Dallman et al., 2004; Rosmond, 2005).

However, time pressure can be viewed as a significant element of work stress, and considerable research points to an association between work stress and unhealthy weight. For example, research in Helsinki found that work fatigue and working overtime were both associated with weight gain among middle-aged employees (Lallukka et al., 2005). A large survey among public sector employees in Finland also found that job stress was associated with higher body mass index (BMI) (Kouvonen et al., 2005). Similarly, an Australian study reported that working long hours was correlated with higher BMI among men (but not women) (Ostry et al., 2006).

Various kinds of stress are known to predict poor health, both physical and mental (Marmot & Wilkinson, 1999). Furthermore, certain disease outcomes associated with stress are also associated with unhealthy weight, suggesting a link between time pressure (as a form of stress) and unhealthy weight. Both psychological and biological mechanisms are involved in these links. There are also plausible biological (metabolic) pathways linking stress and unhealthy weight, particularly abdominal adiposity. Personal coping style may contribute in addition to the disrupted metabolism, resulting in unstable blood sugar (Daniel et al., 1999; McEwen, 1998; Peyrot et al., 1999) and hence unhealthy weight.

In a qualitative study of Australian adults with diabetes, participants reported that working long and irregular hours created difficulties for proper management of their blood sugar levels and weight (Broom, under review; Broom & Whittaker, 2004). Like the Delphi experts, these respondents said that such jobs left them with little time or energy to exercise and made it harder to pay adequate attention to proper diet and cooking. The very phrase 'eating on the run' suggests hurried meals.

Stress, including time pressure, can affect the health of children as well as adults. Canadian and United States cohort studies have found that long hours of parental (especially maternal) employment are associated with excess weight in school age children (Anderson et al., 2003; Phipps et al., forthcoming). A number of mechanisms may be involved: less parental time to walk children to school or to supervise outside play or extracurricular sport, a reliance on fast food, children snacking unsupervised, and parental stress and guilt fostering a tendency to accede to children's demands for energy-dense foods. Stressed parents may themselves engage in comfort eating and may lack the energy for active leisure, thus modelling unhealthy weight-related behaviours to their children. Although they are plausible, there is as yet slender evidence to confirm these proposed connections.

Conclusions

In the absence of an unambiguous cause-and-effect relationship between time pressure and weight, in this chapter we have explored three possibilities. First, we reviewed the evidence that time pressure is increasing, and identified contributors to this increase. Second, it may be that time pressure fosters a rise in population weight in the context of sedentary work and ready access to abundant and appealing energy-dense food. According to this approach, busyness is not inherently a problem for weight, but becomes a problem in the context of calorie abundance and sedentary work, leisure and transport. It is also a problem if, to avoid weight gain, people must allocate extra time for exercise or preparation of less energy-dense food. Third, we considered the limited evidence of associations between time pressure and the health behaviours linked to obesity.

There are, however, other possibilities that we have been unable to evaluate. For example, the link between time pressure and unhealthy weight may be bimodal: people experiencing either too many *or* too few demands on their time may be vulnerable to problems with weight, while people who achieve a balance between their time commitments may also be likely to achieve physical energy balance and hence healthy weight. Finally, perhaps busyness and rising population obesity are not causally related, but they are both complexes or symptoms of modern ways of living. From this perspective, the correlation is spurious, and both are products of modern capitalist materialism and the technological, historical, social and cultural forms that undergird it. We suspect the truth lies in some combination of all these possibilities. A challenging research agenda lies ahead for those who will investigate these important questions.

SIN#3:
THE PRESSURED PARENTING ENVIRONMENT

Parents as piggy in the middle

Cathy Banwell, Megan Shipley and Lyndall Strazdins

Australian children have the dubious honour of coming second only to American children in the weight stakes (Magarey et al., 2003). Childhood overweight and obesity predict the same conditions in adulthood and are associated with increased morbidity and mortality from diseases like diabetes, hypertension and cardiovascular conditions in later life (Caterson, 1999; Dietitians Association of Australia, 2003).

Children, like adults, embody the ills of the modern environment through their increasing weight. They are similarly exposed to a variety of social and cultural influences that operate directly on them as well as through significant people such as peers and parents. This chapter focuses on the cultural and social forces operating on parents to influence the weight of children past weaning age.

Society expects parents to provide children with the basic necessities of life to produce strong, healthy, well-educated citizens. Social, economic and cultural forces bear on parents as they undertake this role. Among them are social norms about 'good parenting', which include appropriate childrearing practices, and the social and economic value and role of children. Ideas about children, their worth and utility are culturally located in time and space, requiring an act of deliberate reflexivity to uncover the pervasive and invisible culture of childrearing at home. Childrearing is a culturally determined activity that reproduces culture over time.

In this chapter we argue that the culture of childrearing establishes relations of power and love between parents and children, and societal expectations of both. More specifically, relationships to food consumption and physical activity are formed by cultural and economic forces such as time restraints on parents and the role of the market in shaping parents' and children's expectations and preferences. Furthermore, structural features such as gender and ethnicity play a role. It is beyond the scope of this chapter to traverse this entire territory, but many of these features are described in chapters by Broom and Strazdins, Smith, and Dixon and Winter.

Expert pressure on parents

Over the last two centuries in America and elsewhere in the developed world, children have lost economic utility and become an economic liability. No longer permitted to provide labour, the role of children now poses a 'tremendous challenge'. It has been accompanied by a shift from the Victorian view of children as 'sturdy innocents' to a 20th-century model of the 'fragile' child requiring 'careful handling or even outright favouritism lest their shaky self-esteem be crushed' (Stearns, 2003, p. 3). The 'challenge' of the role of children is manifested in various guises and contributes to parents' uncertainty in producing these children.

Parenting methods advocated since the 1950s by specialists such as Brazelton, Leach and Spock have set the tone for parenting over this period. Their methods are described as 'child-centred' and 'intensive' (Hays, 1996) in comparison to earlier times (Coveney, 1999; Stearns, 2003). Such methods assume that a parent, usually the mother, will be constantly available to provide for their child's needs. The child is understood as the proper centre of family attention, and it is the child who should *guide* the process of childrearing (Hays, 1996). Although modern childrearing demands unlimited time, patience and a large investment in energy, knowledge and money, it can be seen as a rational response in light of Stearns's observations about modern children's perceived vulnerability. This American joke, sent to the author via email, mocks cultural expectations concerning modern middle-class childrearing, pressures on mothers and failures of fathers.

THE NEXT SURVIVOR SERIES

Six married men will be dropped on an island with one car and three kids each for six weeks. Each kid will play two sports and either take music or dance classes. Each man must take care of his three kids; keep his assigned house clean, correct all homework, complete science projects, cook, do laundry, and pay a list of 'pretend' bills with not enough money.

Each man must also take each child to a doctor's appointment, a dentist appointment and a haircut appointment. He must make one unscheduled and inconvenient visit per child to the Urgent Care (weekend, evening, on a holiday or right when they're about to leave for vacation). He must also make cupcakes for a social function.

Each father will be required to know all of the words to every stupid song that comes on TV and the name of each and every character on cartoons. Each man will have to make an Indian hut model with six toothpicks, a tortilla and one marker; and get a four-year-old to eat a serving of peas. He will need to read a book with the children each night without falling asleep, and then feed them, dress them, brush their teeth and comb their hair each morning by 7:00. They must leave the home with no food on their face or clothes.

The men must try to get through each day without snot, spit-up or barf on their clothing. They must attend weekly school meetings, church, and find time at least once to spend the afternoon at the park or a similar setting. They must clean up after their sick children at 2:00 am and then spend the remainder of the day tending to that child and waiting on them hand and foot until they are better. They must have a loving, age-appropriate reply to 'You're not the boss of me'.

A test will be given at the end of the six weeks, and each father will be required to know all of the following information: each child's birthday, height, weight, shoe size, clothes size and doctor's name. Also the child's weight at birth, length, time of birth, and length of labour, each child's favourite colour, middle name, favourite snack, favourite song, favourite drink, favourite toy, biggest fear and what they want to be when they grow up.

The kids vote them off the island based on performance. The last man wins only if he still has enough energy to be intimate with his spouse at a moment's notice. If the last man does win, he can play the game over and over and over again for the next 18–25 years ... eventually earning the right to be called Mother!

A corollary to the modern approach to childrearing is the rise of the 'democratic rights' of children, which is accompanied by the encouragement of parental indulgence, the almost exclusive responsibility of mothers for children's development, and the possibility through the promise of consumer goods of the indefinite deferral of open conflict with the child. All these are present in much expert advice on parenting, but are also implicit or explicit in advertising to children (Sieter, 1998).

Experts whose words are often amplified and distorted in the popular media have propelled parents towards placing their children at the centre of the household universe and treating them as autonomous individuals. In many cases parents have become increasingly reliant on expert advice with a corresponding loss of confidence in their own judgment about their children's behaviour. Some parents believe that they themselves lack self-control if they intervene in children's behaviour or discipline them (Miller, 2004). Whether this intensive approach has produced the desired confident and capable children is debatable, but it may have had unintended consequences for children's body size. Independent, autonomous children make choices about the food they eat, their social and physical activities, and the products they consume. Parents, having complied with expert advice and societal pressures to produce such autonomous children, are sometimes unable to withdraw or moderate these freedoms when they appear to have negative effects. Parents are then blamed for their children's weight, their behaviour, their psychoses, and sometimes for producing children at all.

Australia and the United States receive expert advice emphasising latitude and autonomy for children while France displays cultural differences in attitudes to children's weight that go back to the 19th century (Stearns, 1999). Throughout the 20th century in America, experts focused on pernickety eaters and underweight children. In contrast, French experts were aware of childhood obesity and emphasised disciplined childhood eating. There was widespread and early acceptance in France that childhood eating should be regulated or controlled. This advice was promoted via pamphlets and courses as part of the 'puericulture campaign'. The campaign noted that children's appetites were a poor guide to feeding and counselled strictly regulated mealtimes. This provides a 'less indulgent picture of childhood in general' in which concerns about underweight were always balanced with greater concern about overweight. Fussy eaters apparently attracted no great interest with the view that if children didn't eat on one day they would eat when they got hungry. These cultural patterns can be seen well past the prime days of the 'puericulture campaigns' with the French still disinclined to snack between meals and showing a general restraint in eating. Stearns argues these cultural differences in the treatment of children and in childhood feeding practices are now entrenched in French culture and embodied so that France has lower levels of population weight than the United States (Stearns, 1999).

Child-centred parenting culture is now more complex. Experts promote the notion that parents should understand children's developmental stages and recognise appropriate behaviour. Parents must move from the flexibility required in feeding infants (see Smith chapter) to establishing age-appropriate boundaries as children develop. Furthermore, parents are exhorted to adopt an 'authoritative' style of parenting which 'reflects positive child guidance, enjoyment in the child, encouragement of child autonomy and affectionate behaviour' (Gable & Lutz, 2000). An authoritarian style which is 'controlling, prohibitive, and anxiety-inducing' should only be used at appropriate times such as 'when a child is running on the street', but parents should encourage 'autonomy at mealtimes' (Gable & Lutz, 2000). Childrearing becomes a daunting task when parents must understand, recognise and conform to this authoritative style while managing children in what are often child-unfriendly environments. Furthermore, parents should harmonise the appropriate style of parenting with their child's physical, social and emotional stage of development. It is not surprising they often do not manage to comply with expert advice.

Piggy in the middle

Research showing children's increased consumption of unhealthy foods such as soft drinks (Gill et al., 2006) and their increasing weight suggests that parents are having difficulties in managing their children's diets. The cultural norms around modern childrearing described above leave parents relatively powerless in the face of children's desires, and the pressures from the marketplace aimed towards encouraging the junior consumer. This book's introduction describes how 50 experts identified changes to parenting practices as one of seven major trends. They specifically described changes in family eating patterns, with children being permitted to eat when and what they liked, as an important trend for childhood obesity (Banwell et al., 2005). Experts noted that children's growing autonomy has allowed them to narrow their food choice to such an extent that their diets are quite restricted, while at the same time their access to food has increased because they can eat whenever they like.

Research shows that young children innately prefer energy-dense foods such as dairy products or foods that are sweet or starchy (Cooke, 2004) and that attempts to control children's diets or pressure children to eat healthy foods using rewards, punishment or providing health information are unsuccessful (Fisher, 1999). Another view suggests that children are 'food neophobic' (afraid of new foods) and are naturally suspicious of fruit and vegetables. Parents respond to this by attempting to control their diets (Cooke, 2004). Even if, as some studies argue, children can self-regulate their food intake when only nutritious food is available, they are unlikely to do so when highly desirable, less healthy snack foods are offered (Schwartz & Puhl, 2003). To modify children's diets parents are advised to repeatedly expose their young children to healthier foods to overcome their innate fear of new (healthy) foods (Schwartz & Puhl, 2003; Wardle et al., 2003) and set a good example with their own eating patterns (Cooke, 2004), but few parents are aware of this.

We argue instead that children exert a powerful influence on family eating patterns, which is exploited by (TV) advertisers. In the United States, an important opportunity for socialising children and developing their values, the family meal, is being replaced by TV viewing while dining, which promotes 'materialistic attitudes' (Marquis, 2004). A United Kingdom report identified television viewing as a key factor in childhood obesity. Time spent watching TV correlates with poor diet, poor health and obesity among both children and adults. The authors offered three explanations for the association: TV viewing is sedentary, it is associated with snacking, and it is linked with the consumption of pre-prepared and convenience foods (Livingstone & Helsper, 2004). Australian children who spend more than two hours a day watching television are likely to eat significantly more snack foods and high energy drinks, eat less fruit, and are less likely to participate in organised physical activity (Salmon et al., 2006). These arguments receive greater attention in the chapter by Dugdale and Dixon.

External pressures on children to consume particular foods influence parental food purchasing and preparation. Men have been displaced from the 19th-century vision as the 'head of the table' mirroring a shift from 'father to breadwinner' (Williams, 2000). A study among Melbourne adults on the place of chicken meat consumption within the family diet (Dixon, 2002) illustrates how children's food preferences have a major impact on family eating (Dixon & Banwell, 2004).

The heightened influence of children on the family diet illustrates the importance of expert advice on feeding children. 'Parents actively seek out expert advice about the "proper way" of raising children ... They do it as a way of bringing about their ethical completion as parents' (Coveney, 1999). The importance of fostering dietary freedom and independence in children is explicit in the recommendations of contemporary nutritionists. Food needs to be 'enjoyable' and family eating should promote happiness and harmony. Parents are also urged to negotiate with children to ensure their diet is healthy, which involves juggling children's autonomy and their happiness (Coveney, 1999).

One way this is accomplished is through parental labour, usually that of mothers. They sometimes cook and serve several meals at a time, one for adults and another for children. Coveney interviewed a father who claimed that his son is spoilt by his mother and grandmother. 'He [son] quite often gets different things cooked for him because he doesn't like this and he doesn't like that' (Coveney, 1999, p. 270). Mothers are exhorted in parenting magazines and books on feeding children to encourage children to eat healthy foods by making food that is colourful and fun, sometimes in the form of a visual image such as a face or a boat. They are instructed to include children in food preparation and cooking so they will learn to see food as enjoyable although doing so is often time consuming and messy, demanding considerable parental time and effort. The number of books and magazine articles devoted to advising parents on how to feed their children points to the high anxiety around this topic.

The time squeeze: Mothers' work pressures and children's weight

To be seen as a 'good mother', women should devote unlimited amounts of love, time, patience and physical labour to the wellbeing of their children (Boulton, 1983; Brown et al., 1997; Lupton & Fenwick, 2001). The ideology of intensive mothering, in which mothering is made sacred, results in mothers feeling uncomfortable or unable to delegate childrearing. The normative domestic arrangement that identifies women as carers and men as breadwinners turns labour into love. Women stay home to care for children but – 'they happen to pick up the dry cleaning and clean the toilets as well' (Williams, 2000).

This places mothers at the centre of contradictory cultural, economic and social trends (Hays, 1996). Pressures on women to define themselves by their non-maternal activities have been growing (Lupton, 2000) despite the increased expectations associated with intensive mothering (Hays, 1996). Delphi study experts identified paid work as a significant pressure on parents, particularly women, constraining their time and energy for other activities. Over the last 50 years women's involvement in the paid economy has increased and been affected by growing demands for casual labour and long or 'unsociable' working hours (see the chapter by Broom and Strazdins). Domestic arrangements where both partners in a marriage now work has increased over the last five years and currently stands at 43 per cent of all families with children aged less than 15 years (Australian Bureau of Statistics, 2003a) but men still spend less time in domestic work and women perform more childcare than men (Bittman, 1999).

Recently we examined the relationship between children's body mass index (BMI) and mothers' working hours and pressured work conditions. The study conducted in the Australian Capital Territory (ACT), contained 175 working mothers with 305 children aged 5 to seventeen. Seventy-three mothers worked in the retail industry, 69 in the public service and a further 32 were employed partners of men who worked in one of these industries. A similar proportion of women were overweight to Australian general population (see table 1) (Cameron et al., 2003). As in other studies (Strauss & Knight, 1999), mothers and children's BMIs were positively correlated.

TABLE 1 Weights of mothers and children in the ACT work and health study

	Normal weight %	Just overweight %	Overweight %	Obese %
ACT work & health mothers	48	na	29	22
ACT work & health children	68	17	11	na
Australian general population	48	na	30	22

We grouped children's consumption of foods in the preceding 24 hours into few or many serves of healthy (for example, fruit and vegetables) and unhealthy foods. The children of mothers who worked only standard hours or had a regular work schedule were significantly more likely to eat more serves of healthy foods in the preceding 24 hours.

As mothers' work hours, job demands and job insecurity increased, so did children's BMI. In contrast, as mothers' work rewards and control over their jobs increased, children's BMIs decreased.

A scale was constructed of positive working conditions (the Job Quality Index), including family friendly workplace, sociable work hours, flexible work hours, job control, job security, a supportive work environment, low levels of work conflict, and a feasible workload. The more positive job qualities mothers reported, the lower the BMI of their children. However, mothers' reports that their time with their children was limited, the amount of support they got in the workplace and conflict between their work and social demands were not correlated with children's BMI. Mothers with higher job control and greater work rewards had lower BMIs, and so did their children.

As we expected, children's BMIs were lower among higher socioeconomic status (SES) parents. But all correlations between work conditions and children's BMI, with the exception of job control, remained after controlling for SES. Thus, while SES is important it did not over-ride the other factors. This is in contrast to North American studies where the main associations with children's BMI have been with socioeconomic variables such as parents' income (Gable & Lutz, 2000), maternal education and parental education (Strauss & Knight, 1999). In one study mothers' hours worked per week were associated with increased BMI in children only for children from high income families with well-educated mothers (Anderson et al., 2003).

Academic commentators have expressed concern about the contribution of convenience and pre-prepared food to unhealthy weight of adults and children. Ethnographic studies show that convenience foods are accepted because they are perceived to offer solutions to the organisation of everyday life. In the early part of the 20th century convenience was about making life more comfortable; now it is about the reordering of time. Convenience 'relaxes the constraints upon an individual's trajectory through time and space' (Warde et al., 1998). Convenience foods are considered quick and easy; foods that 'you don't have to think about' (Banwell et al., 2005) thus saving mental as well as physical energy. They continue to grow in popularity. Between 1984 and 1994, the proportion of the Australian household budget spent on eating out and takeaway food and beverages increased by 5 per cent to 23 per cent (Australian Bureau of Statistics, 1998). Convenience foods are associated with growing obesity because they are energy dense with a high fat content (Prentice & Jebb, 2003), portions are often large and they can be consumed anytime and anywhere. They are easily carried, can be eaten on the run, and often don't require cutlery. Their nutrient content is often hidden so that consumers relinquish control over what they are eating (Prentice & Jebb, 2003).

Recent research points to intervening factors within the family. For example, a Canadian study found that children have lower BMIs if families regularly eat meals together. Such children, opined the authors, have healthier diets, are less likely to be 'mindlessly eating' in front of television and may also benefit from better communication and interaction with their parents (Veugelers & Fitzgerald, 2005). In a United States study children who eat family dinners were less likely to eat ready-made food (Gillman et al., 2000). In Australia, the importance of mothers' positive attitudes towards family dining was found to have more impact on maintaining children's healthy weight than self-reports of the family eating together (Mamun et al., 2005).

Overall, though, time shortage and pressures resulting from poor job quality may leave mothers with little opportunity or energy to monitor children's food intake, prepare family meals, restrict children's screen viewing, and encourage outdoor or active play. These factors, implicated in childhood obesity, are characterised as 'parental under-control' (Gable & Lutz, 2000).

The money squeeze: Financial pressures on children's physical activities

Thus far we have argued that children's weight is influenced by cultural pressures on parents to indulge their children's desires to consume. But what about parents who are not in a financial position to do this?

Research is now focusing on the relationship between children's activities and childhood obesity. We extend this by considering the financial barriers to children's activities. Although this has not been explored thoroughly, there is evidence to suggest that financial pressures on parents limit their children's activities. This may contribute to higher obesity levels among low SES groups due to less physical and intellectual stimulation (Strauss & Knight, 1999) (see also the Dugdale and Dixon chapter). This mother's statement exemplifies how an expanded income would increase her children's activities:

> Oh well, I'd take the kids on more outings. We'd go on more holidays. They'd have already been to the zoo if I had money. They would have already seen certain things. (Banwell & Bammer, unpublished)

As yet, no Australian published research examines the costs of children's physical activities in light of obesity trends. At present there is no consensus on estimating the costs of raising children. Rather than engaging in debates about methods for estimating the costs of raising children in Australia (Percival & Harding, 2005; Saunders, 1999) we list the costs of activities in which ACT-based school age children known to the lead author, participate.

Their activities are described in light of the findings from a United Kingdom paper on children's calorific expenditures on activities (Mackett et al., 2005). That study monitored 10–13-year-old children's activities and examined differences between school-based activities, structured and unstructured out-of-home events and travel. It defines a structured event as one in which children's activities are determined by an adult, while an unstructured event is one where the child determines the type and level of activity. It also includes a range of out-of-home events shared with parents.

It found that activities outside the home use more calories than activities inside the home. Being at home had the second lowest level of activity after being in school lessons. 'Only 10 per cent of children's time spent at their own home is of moderate or higher intensity, despite the fact that this includes playing in the garden' (Mackett et al., 2005). Unstructured out-of-home events had significantly higher levels of activity intensity than structured out-of home activities. Furthermore, children were more likely to walk to them while they were usually chauffeured to structured events. Walking was second only to physical education and games in its calorific intensity.

Out-of-home activity uses more calories than being at home (Mackett et al., 2005), so we priced a range of 'out-of-home events shared with parents'. It costs a family $69 to visit the National Zoo and Aquarium in the ACT: children aged 4–15 pay $12.50 (concessions are available) and adults pay $23.50. Another special family event in Canberra is a visit to the annual show. In 2006, a family entry ticket for two adults and two children was $38, with any further child costing $8. One Canberra family consisting of two adults and three children estimated that they spent approximately $200 on their day at the show, which included one or two rides per child, one show bag, and some show food, petrol and parking costs. When discussing the cost, a parent commented that it is hardly possible to attend the show and refuse children one ride and one show bag at least. A trip to the circus, another summer entertainment in Canberra in 2006, was $112 per family of four. The price of an adult ticket was $46 but $32 if receiving a concession and $22 per child. Even a trip to the pictures costs $15 for adults and $9 for children; $48 for the family. Such events according to the Mackett study fall in the mid-range of activity intensity.

There are of course less expensive and more physically intense activities on offer. For example, a two-hour session at an ice skating rink costs $12 plus $3 for skate hire. Indoor rock climbing costs $12 per student, with additional costs for hire of harnesses, chalk bags and shoes. Swimming pools are cheaper with costs of around $5 per adult and around $2 to $3 for children. Pools have the additional advantage of not requiring the hire of special gear. But as one single mother commented, a trip to the pool will cost well over $10 because you have to buy ice-creams. An hour's trail ride at local horse riding schools will cost $20 to $30 per person.

Structured out-of-home events, such as sports participation, use slightly fewer calories than unstructured ones (Mackett et al., 2005). Costs associated with a range of these types of activities generally require an up-front payment for club membership and equipment that may be prohibitive to many families. For a child to play soccer, which is the fastest growing boy's sport attracting 19.6 per cent of the non-adult male population (Australian Bureau of Statistics, 2003b), costs $110 plus uniform and boots. Netball is the most popular girls' sport in Australia with 18.2 per cent of the non-adult female population participating (Australian Bureau of Statistics, 2003b). A season of netball costs between $60 and $85 per child depending on their age, with an additional $11 for club affiliation, plus the costs of uniform and special shoes. If children play a summer and winter sport, the costs approximately double per year. The ACT, which is on average an affluent area, has fairly high rates of participation in organised sport with 70 per cent of boys and 54.6 per cent of girls aged 5–14 participating (Australian Bureau of Statistics, 2003b). No data is available that correlates children's participation and socioeconomic status. However, 40 per cent of children from families in which no adult is employed participate in organised sport, while 81 per cent of children with two employed parents participate.

A full year's membership of scouts (now for girls and boys) in one of the Canberra clubs is $240. Additional activities, such as camps and outings are not included in these fees. There is also an increasing trend towards children's birthday parties and group gatherings being held at commercial establishments, with costs of at least $8 to $15 per child.

Unstructured out-of-home events include ball games (for example, kicking a football) and activities such as cycling, scootering, skateboarding and general play. Sixty-two per cent of Australian children aged 5–14 spent an average of six hours over a school fortnight and 23 per cent skateboarded or rollerbladed for five hours per school fortnight (Australian Bureau of Statistics,

2003b). These activities are free but require equipment such as skateboards, bikes or scooters, which can be bought cheaply second-hand but are expensive if purchased new. For example, a small child's bike or trike can cost anything between $30 and $80, but once children need a large bike prices rapidly reach $300 or more for a new one. Cheaper ones are available through chain stores, but if they break, some cycle shops will not repair them because they are considered of inferior quality.

Delphi participants (Banwell & Bammer, unpublished) noted the replacement of unstructured activities by screen-based play at home and attributed it to a number of changes in Australians' lives, such as the fears for children's safety when outside, and loss of playing spaces due to urban and housing design (see the chapter by Dugdale and Dixon). Accumulating evidence associates environmental design of higher SES neighbourhoods with increasing adult levels of physical activities (Ball et al., 2001; Kavanagh et al., 2005). Over time, wild spaces have been developed and such areas have become less accessible. Because they are less likely to live near beaches, rivers, parks and playing fields, children from poorer families are more likely to experience loss of playing space than those from wealthier families.

Parents worry about their children's safety. They cite fear of traffic accidents and 'stranger danger' as reasons for not letting children walk to school or play outside. Parents from more disadvantaged areas frequently perceive their suburb to be dangerous and restrict their children's movements (Palmer et al., 2005). Fear of crime, bullying and stranger danger were cited in one lower SES New Zealand suburb (Whittenet al., 2003). Such fears may be internalised so that a child seen outside by itself is considered a sign of bad parenting. In areas where drug use is common, fear of needle-stick injuries is an additional reason to restrict younger children's outdoor play. Older children are often perceived to be dangerous to others and their non-structured activities, such as skateboarding, become subject to control by local authorities and disapproval from adults (Nolan, 2003).

The costs of school activities also exclude children from participating. This Canberra single mother receiving a disability pension commented:

Some weeks I've just gotten by and other weeks, I haven't. Well, the worst week I had was when my son's school camp was on and I had to pay for the school camp and all that sort of stuff. (Banwell, 2003)

Qualitative research conducted in Melbourne indicates that low incomes families there have similar concerns. Parents raised the issues of school camp ($240), school shoes and other school expenses, travel to sporting competitions and dance classes (Taylor, 2004). In 2006 it cost $230 for children at a Canberra public school to attend Year 6 camp, which is less expensive than previous years after parents complained about the costs.

To participate in many of the activities we have described, such as team sports, requires a car in a car-reliant society such as Australia. However, Mackett et al. (2005) argue that in the United Kingdom walking, particularly to school, is the most energy-expending calorific form of exercise children undertake. Car ownership is associated with lower likelihood of walking among adults (Carlin et al., 1997) and thus one would expect that lower car ownership levels among poorer families should reduce the chances of obesity among their children.

Despite the likelihood of living in a car-owning family, children living in medium and high SES areas are more likely to walk to school if they are aged 5–6 and even more so if they are aged 10–12 (Timperio et al., 2006). A survey of students at a primary school in a middle-class suburb in the ACT showed that 26 per cent of children walked to and from school, 5.8 per cent cycled, 65 per cent travelled in a car or taxi and 2.6 per cent caught a bus (Aranda Primary School, 2006). At present we do not know whether children from a low SES family without a car maintain a healthy weight. However, carlessness may mean that children miss out on so many family and school activities that this overwhelms the health benefits of alternative transport use (see Hinde chapter). Financially pressured car-owning families may not have discretionary income to spend on children's activities. These children may also experience many of the environmental deterrents to walking to school associated with less affluent neighbourhoods (Timperio et al., 2006). Considering the interaction of car-use and financial resources begs a question:

What role will increasing petrol costs in Australia have in influencing children's weights?

Researchers identify a psychosocial component to poverty and non-participation. In the United Kingdom it was found that transport and participation costs leave children on the periphery of social and leisure experience, as this boy describes:

> I would like to do more things with my friends, when they go out down the town and that. But we can't always afford it. So I got to stay in and that, and just in here it's just boring – I can't do anything. (Mike, 12 years) (cited in Ridge, 2003)

And this girl limits her activities rather than face the judgment of her peers:

> You can't do as much, and I don't like my clothes and that. So I don't really get to do much or do stuff like friends are doing ... I'm worried about what people will think of me, like they think I'm sad [pathetic] or something. (Nicole, 13 years) (cited in Ridge, 2003)

Both quotations illustrate how poverty can lead to physical inactivity, to 'staying in'. For poorer people, the social discomfort and financial costs of activities may compare unfavourably with the comfort of screen-based forms of entertainment at home. Low income households usually contain TVs and DVD or video players. They provide inexpensive entertainment for all members of the family once their initial purchase cost is covered. For special occasions, the hire of a DVD at $6 that can be watched by as many people as a room can accommodate is much cheaper than a family participating in more active entertainments.

'Consumption is an important mechanism for constructing and signalling social relationships between parents and children, between family and non-family members' (Clarke, 2003). Even when money is scarce, many parents will strive for social and cultural reasons to satisfy children's urge to consume and to participate in a consuming peer group. Poorer parents are less likely to spend money on activities that demand a large upfront financial commitment, or that require major on-going expenses. Cigarette consumption, although expensive and unhealthy in the long run, is a relatively accessible and affordable pleasure or stress relief for those with little money. Screen-based activities and unhealthy foods may fulfil a similar role for children.

Conclusion

In light of declining population levels in Australia, and concerns about the demographic constitution of the Australian population, the Treasurer Peter Costello in 2005 famously exhorted couples 'to have one [child] for the mother, one for the father and one for the country'. Here the role of children is to provide pleasure and fulfilment for their parents. The most attention grabbing part of this statement, however, was the instruction to have 'one for the country', suggesting that it is children's role to replenish population stocks presumably to support ageing baby-boomers (including the Treasurer) and reproduce mainstream Australian culture or the 'Australian way of life'.

In this chapter we have argued that parents are not solely responsible for their children's weight. They and their children are caught in an obesogenic environment that is itself the product of cultural, social and economic trends many of which are promulgated by the marketplace and by government. The Treasurer sees children as an investment, while the Health Minister indicates that overweight children are an economic liability. Such disparate political views need to be harmonised to work on the many features of children's obesogenic environment that policy-makers can influence. These include controls on marketing, advertising and product placement, management of the interaction between work and care environments to provide parents with time and energy to spend with their children, and ensuring that children have access to a wide range of intellectually stimulating physical and outdoor activities irrespective of their social and economic position. While current contradictory economic and social forces operate on parents in the early 21st century, it is unlikely that trends in children's obesity will be reversed rapidly.

SIN#4:
THE TECHNOLOGICAL ENVIRONMENT

Digital technologies or space to play (up) and belong?

Anni Dugdale and Jane Dixon

A great deal of social research portrays young people as a problem. Youth culture has long been depicted as a threat to the mainstream (Parsons, 1964). Living in a world characterised by risk and uncertainty (Beck, 1992) can heighten fears that children and young people will not be up to the task of running things when their turn comes (Butcher & Thomas, 2003). Today these intergenerational fears are increasingly being represented as located in young people's immersion in the electronic media – playing computer games, surfing the Net and watching TV. There is a widespread discourse in which parents struggle with the latest in home computing, while their children readily adapt and innovate using a range of new technologies – gameboys, playstations, the Internet, TVs in every room, DVD and MP3 players, mobile phones and SMS. Worrying about children and young people's use of digital technologies has become routine.

Most recently, these worries have come to focus on fears that the digital age has contributed to the overall epidemic of overweight and obesity. Several Australian summits and taskforces in the last few years have targeted obesity: the National Health and Medical

Research Council Strategic Plan for Prevention of Overweight and Obesity (National Health and Medical Research Centre, 1997), the NSW Obesity Summit (NSW Department of Health, 2003; Devlin, 2004), the National Obesity Taskforce (National Obesity Taskforce, 2003), and the launch of 'Building a healthy and active Australia' (www.healthyactive.gov.au/internet/healthyactive/publishing.nsf/Content/home 2004).

Rising population rates of obesity and overweight are perceived as a consequence of economic growth, greater affluence and increased consumption (see the Denniss chapter). The bodies of children and young people, we are told, are being reshaped by the postmodern digital age. Rapid increases in the rates of overweight and obesity among children and adolescents are being blamed on screen-related sedentary behaviour.

Media spotlight on childhood obesity

This is certainly the story that is being broadcast by the popular media. 'Children particularly spend a lot more time playing computer games, watching television, and eating fatty snacks … instead of playing outdoors' ('Fighting fat kids: fat chance', ABC Radio National, 'Health Matters', March 2003). The world where children now grow up was described in a recent ABC 'Four Corners' documentary 'Generation O' (O being for obesity) as 'toxic, pathological and obesogenic'. The program opened with shots of children and young people at a local suburban shopping mall, hanging out and eating fast foods. The camera lingered on those who were fat, and the voice-over drew the audience's attention to the fact that one in four Australian children are overweight or obese (ABC TV, 'Four Corners', 17 October 2005).

Proportions of overweight and obese children and young people reported in the media vary from one-fifth to two-thirds, but whatever the figures quoted they are described as an epidemic, a disaster, a crisis. Radio broadcasters lament the passing of the time when 'backyards rang to the sound of balls being booted and whacked', now deserted by children much more likely to be inside at the Playstation, TV or Internet ('Where do the children play?' ABC Radio National, 'Health Matters', April 2005). This theme is also reflected in the print media. The *Sydney Morning Herald*, reporting results from a number of ongoing child health studies at the beginning of 2005, set the scene by comparing today's children who 'spend too much time playing computer games' with the active childhoods of the past where children freely roamed their neighbourhoods, 'hanging out in cubbyhouses, digging holes, and playing in the creek' ('What kids really want', *SMH*, 2 February 2005).

Computer games are rarely blamed as the sole culprit, but they nevertheless take centre stage. The message from public health professionals and researchers that the causes of increased rates of obesity and overweight in children and young people are multiple and interactive *is* part of the popular media's storyline. Like the broadcast media programs cited above, the *Sydney Morning Herald* is typical when it declares that 'There are many villains in the puzzle. They include TV and computer games, fast food and advertising, lack of exercise and the car loving society' ('What kids really want', *SMH*, 2 February 2005). But screen time, and particularly playing computer and video games, has become emblematic.

Counteracting excessive screen time by encouraging more physical activity became the jumping off point for government policy in 2006. The Federal Government launched a $6 million 'Get Moving' campaign to encourage children to exercise for at least one hour a day (www.healthyactive.gov.au/). The message to parents emphasises that children 'should not spend more than two hours a day using electronic media for entertainment (for example, computer games, TV, Internet)'. Notably absent from the policy were any curbs to food and drink advertising on children's television, curbs supported by the then Opposition Leader Mark Latham. Indeed, Prime Minister John Howard lambasted such proposals as 'a stupid, ill-conceived ban' and backed 'choices' about the family diet being clearly an area of parental responsibility where governments did not belong. In launching the 'Get Moving' campaign, Health Minister Tony Abbott reiterated this viewpoint: 'We are a free people in a free country and the last thing I want to do is start dictating the menu in every Australian home, dictating what appears on every Australian television' (*Herald Sun*, 4 February 2006).

To target children and young people and to criticise their leisure time choices is much less politically sensitive than advertising bans. However, it could be argued that criticising the youth and children of Australia and their parents for living out the high consumption, high technology dream is unlikely to bring about a return to the active leisure time pursuits of earlier generations, whether that is cricket or netball, or the slightly more contemporary and free-wheeling activities of swimming, basketball, handball and dancing. These are the activities portrayed in the 'Get Moving' television advertising aimed at the 40 per cent of Australian children who do not participate in organised sports.

The remainder of this chapter explores the extent to which the activity patterns of children and young people changed over the previous two decades. Can the new digital leisure pursuits of postmodern society be blamed for rising rates of obesity and overweight among children and young people? And perhaps more importantly, if it is vital to reverse the trends in obesity and overweight among children and young people, how can that happen in ways that do not increase the burden of disadvantage and stigma so easily attached to children who are overweight?

Weight worries about the young

Before child and adolescent rates of obesity and overweight became a regular feature in the popular media, they were first researched and reported in the health literature. Here the story was more nuanced and more carefully told, but still viewed with alarm.

Trends in overweight and obesity for children and young people parallel those for Australian adults, but nevertheless should be differentiated from them. Based on the 1995 ABS National Nutrition Survey, 18.3 per cent of boys and 16.9 per cent of girls aged 10–14 are overweight and 4.1 per cent of boys and 4.9 per cent of girls are obese (Australian Institute of Health and Welfare, 2004). Even allowing for increases in the decade to 2005, these figures are markedly lower than for Australian adults and the actual population numbers are not in the same league as they are for adults (see the chapter by Friel and Broom). However, the rates of increase are significant and, as with adults, it is important to note that the increased frequency of overweight and obesity is not spread evenly across all groups of children and young people. The level of combined overweight–obesity in children doubled for both boys and girls aged 12–15 and for girls but not boys aged 7–12 in the decade to 1995 (Magarey et al. 2001). The level of obesity trebled for both boys and girls aged 7–15 between 1985 and 1997 (Booth et al. 2003, p. 29). This was a far sharper rise than experienced in the previous 16 years (1969–85), when for girls the prevalence of combined overweight and obesity did not alter, although for boys the combined level increased in those years by 60 per cent (Booth et al., 2003, p. 29). According to a new study conducted by the NSW Centre for Overweight and Obesity, rates of overweight and obesity have continued to rise, with 7–15 year old males being at particular risk. For the first time, the percentage of overweight/obese boys in that age bracket surpasses that for girls (Robotham, 2006).

Being an overweight child is not a strong predictor of being an overweight adult; three in four overweight children will not go on to become overweight adults (Skidmore & Yarnel, 2004; Venn & Dwyer, 2005; Wright et al., 2001). However, according to one very large Norwegian study that followed up 14–19 year olds for 31 years, being an overweight adolescent carries a risk of premature death (Engeland et al., 2003).

With the tenuous relationship between childhood obesity and adult obesity, why is there such a strong focus on children as the target of interventions to reduce unhealthy weight? Reasons put forward to make children and adolescents a national priority include the following (Australian Institute of Health and Welfare, 2005; Booth et al., 2003; Lobstein et al., 2004; Skidmore & Yarnel, 2004):

- The accelerating rates of obesity and overweight in this age group in the last decade could be an indicator of future adult rates continuing to climb alarmingly.
- Eating and activity patterns established early in life are persistent across the lifespan, and even children who are not yet overweight may carry a poor balance of eating and activity patterns into adult life leading to later onset of obesity.

- Poor health outcomes, particularly onset of type 2 diabetes, are rising rapidly and for the first time ever becoming prevalent amongst children and young people as a result of declines in activity levels and weight gain.

It is not merely the known additional health risks burdening the 5 per cent of obese children (aged 2–14 years) that is driving this new public health agenda (Botero & Wolfsdorf, 2005; Dunstan et al., 2002; Lobstein et al., 2004). Some researchers admit that the focus on children is motivated by a perception that it is easier to change children's behaviour because they are more likely to be closely supervised (Lobstein et al., 2004), and their behaviour is thought to be more subject to control than that of adults.

Activity patterns and trends among young people

State-based studies indicate that the majority of children and adolescents meet the one hour a day physical activity guideline, although participation rates are consistently lower for females and they decline for both sexes with increasing years. However, a sizable proportion of adolescents (one-quarter to one-third) do less than the recommended daily amount of activity (Australian Bureau of Statistics, 2006).

For all the attention being paid to the dangers of modern childhood, remarkably little is known about generational changes in activity patterns and preferences. So estimating even crude trends requires a synthesising approach to assembling available pieces of evidence from a range of sources, including routine data collections, one-off and repeat surveys and intervention studies.

The most studied technology in obesity research is the television. Australian Bureau of Statistics (ABS) data indicate that in 2000 all houses had at least one television, with 61 per cent containing more than one. TV was introduced in Australia in 1956, and was an expensive luxury. In less than 50 years, Australian children have come to spend a median of 160 minutes per day watching television (Olds et al., 2006). The advent of television spawned other possibilities for watching movies at home, courtesy of the video recorder (VCR). The making of 'home entertainment', a term synonymous with TV and related technologies, means that families no longer have to expend energy leaving the house to see movies but 'can sit back and relax' not far from the fridge and pantry. The uptake of VCRs has been dramatic, rising from 3 per cent in 1981 to 86 per cent in 2000, allowing the vast majority of households to be passively entertained at all times, every day.

The 24/7 capability of TV viewing has been complemented by another technology that can encroach on the time available for active pursuits or for sleep. As recently as 1985, only a tiny percentage of Australian households contained a computer, but 15 years later about half of all homes had one. With computer access has come a blossoming of possibilities for entertainment while sitting down: Internet access rose from 4 per cent in 1996 to over 24 per cent of households in 2000, half of which contain children between 5 and 14 years of age. Understandably, some worry that 'increased accessibility to television and computers is likely to have resulted in increased levels of sedentary behaviour in children' (Olds et al., 2004). Certainly time spent watching television has increased for Australian children from 113 minutes per day in 1992 to 130 minutes per day in 1997 (ABS, 1997) to the 160 minutes noted above for South Australian children aged 10–13 years, at least (Olds et al., 2006). Other screen-based activities have also increased, with Internet usage rising for both boys (48 per cent in 2000 to 62 per cent in 2003) and girls (46 per cent to 66 per cent in corresponding years) (ABS, 2006).

In the South Australian study conducted in 2002 (one of the very few studies to consider time spent in front of television, video games and the computer), median total screen time was found to be 229 minutes per day varying from 264 minutes for boys to 196 minutes for girls (Olds et al., 2006, p. 139). While this is almost double the recommended daily allocation to such activities, the associations between body mass index (BMI) category and screen time were observed but not significant. Using a 1959–60 study of Perth children's out-of-school activities to compare with a 2003 ABS survey of children's leisure time, Carter (2005) argued that the amount of time children allocated to television/video had declined by 33 minutes between 1960 and 2003. When the amount of time they now spent on computers/electronic games was included in sedentary activity, Carter concluded that the amount of sedentary time that Perth children spent on digital activities had barely changed in the intervening 43 years.

Apportioning blame to digital technologies becomes tricky when one looks for evidence of how screen-based activities have displaced other activities that involve greater levels of energy expenditure (Palmer, 1986), although a few studies are beginning to show that this is happening. For example, it appears that when TV viewing becomes a preferred leisure activity among primary school girls, they are less inclined to be physically active (Salmon, Timperio, Cleland, & Venn, 2005a). And for South Australian boys and girls, a relationship has been shown between high screen use and reductions in sport and play and in sleep, and a decrease in moderate to vigorous physical activity (Olds et al., 2006, p. 139).

The evidence is most equivocal concerning whether the progressive introduction of electronic and digital technologies has been at the expense of participation in organised sport (at club or school). Nationally, the latest ABS data show that 62 per cent of 5–14 year olds participated in organised sport in their free time in 2003 (ABS, 2006), with a small drop in girls' sports participation between 2000–03, although their involvement in cultural activities (music, dancing, singing and drama) outside of school increased from 40 per cent to 43 per cent. For boys, there was a drop in cultural activities participation: 20 per cent to 17 per cent.

Perhaps community concerns about child health have already arrested declines in physical activity, if a 2004 New South Wales survey of Year 8 and Year 10 students is any guide. That survey revealed a 26 per cent increase in at least one hour of moderate or vigorous activity among girls since 1997, and a 30 per cent increase among boys. Boys' greater weight rise alongside their increased physical activity prompted one newspaper caption to read, 'fitter and fatter', with experts implicating dietary intake as the major culprit (Robotham, 2006).

Although physical activity rates among children and adolescents may have fluctuated in the last 20 years, it is instructive to note children's changing preferences for how they like to spend out-of-school hours. Surveys conducted since 1957 that have asked children to nominate their favourite ways of using leisure time suggest that:

- while playing sport remains popular, television viewing has shown a rapid rise in popularity from being ranked thirteenth for boys in 1974 to number four in 2000, and rising from tenth to second most popular for girls in the same period;
- eating and sleeping have recently appeared for the first time in the top ten preferred leisure activities;
- there is a shift away from traditional organised sports like cricket and tennis toward newer sports like basketball and aerobics which 'may represent a trend toward "take away" sports which require less time commitment (training and matchplay)' (Olds et al., 2004, p. 23); and
- in 1994 boys and girls listed seven 'active' pursuits in their top ten, compared to two to three for boys and three to four for girls in 2000 (Olds et al., 2004, p. 45).

In short, there is a consistent trend toward favouring passive leisure over active leisure. However, the epidemiological literature cannot establish how much of the rise of overweight and obesity is caused by any single fad in physical activity, including the ubiquity of computer and video games in the lives of children and young people. In a recent comprehensive review of the internationally available data, conflicting evidence about the nature and impact of TV watching in long-term studies of national populations was documented (Dollman et al., 2005).

Some investigations of screen-based activity patterns have found little association with weight gain, possibly because few studies consider the range of screen-based activities. Using Australian data collected from almost 3000 school children, Wake and colleagues (2003) reported no relationship between electronic games and child BMI, but they did find a relationship with TV viewing time. In contrast, United States panel study data with over 3000 participants failed to show any association between children's weight status and TV viewing but did find a curvilinear relationship between electronic games use and weight status for children under 8 years of age. Children with lower weight played electronic games for either very little or very large amounts of time, with heavier children spending moderate amounts of time playing electronic games (Vandewater et al., 2004). Other studies do, however, confirm the findings from Wake and colleagues concerning an association between time spent watching TV and overweight (Andersen, 2000; Sekine et al., 2002), especially for children with TVs in their bedrooms (Dennison et al., 2002).

The cross-sectional nature of most research can only reveal associations between television viewing habits and childhood obesity risk factors (namely, physical activity, diet and sleep), rather than a direct relationship to the onset of obesity. In a large Melbourne-based study, children who watched more than two hours of television a day were more likely than their peers who watched less than this amount to: have one or more serves per day of high energy drinks; have one or more servings per day of savoury snacks; consume fewer than two or more serves of fruit; or not participate in organised physical activity (Salmon et al., 2006). A number of studies report findings of an association between hours spent watching television and lower levels of activity and energy-dense diet consumption (Andersen, 2000; Francis et al., 2003; Giammattei et al., 2003; Goldberg et al., 1978). Confirmation of the overall association between television viewing and weight rise has come most recently from a suite of studies reported in the *Archives of Pediatrics & Adolescent Medicine*. The reported findings included: a) preschoolers who watch more than two hours of TV a day were at risk of overweight (Lumeng et al., 2006); b) children's screen media exposure is a prospective risk factor for children's requests for advertised products, especially food/drinks (Chamberlain et al., 2006); and c) in a two-year follow-up study of children (mean age of 11.6 years at baseline), each hourly increase in television viewing was associated with an extra 167 kilocaleries per day, due to increased consumption of foods commonly advertised on TV (Wiecha et al., 2006).

Time lags between measuring the behaviour and observing health effects are required to attribute causal relationships. Two longitudinal studies have examined the impact of excessive television viewing in childhood and later overweight. Following a group of 1000 New Zealanders from birth in 1972 and 1973 until they were 26 years, researchers found that average weeknight viewing between ages 5–15 was associated with higher BMI at age

26, lower cardio-respiratory fitness, higher serum cholesterol and increased cigarette smoking. These associations persisted after adjustment for childhood socioeconomic status (SES) and a range of other factors, including physical activity at age 15 years. The researchers attributed 17 per cent of the overweight in 26 year olds to watching more than two hours a day of TV during childhood and adolescence (Hancox et al., 2004). Analyses of the 1958 British birth cohort study reveal a less straightforward picture. BMI and physical activity frequency were recorded at 11, 16, 23, 33 and 42 years and television frequency at 11, 16 and 23 years. Women who watched TV most frequently at 11 years and both sexes at 23 years had higher BMIs. However, BMI and television viewing were unrelated for 11-year-old males and for 16-year-old boys and girls, leading to the conclusion that BMI, physical activity and television viewing change with age (Parsons et al., 2005), and may differ by gender.

It appears to us that it is premature to attribute children's physical activity and attendant high BMI, at least for girls, to digital technologies. The evidence is more solid in relation to linking TV viewing and consumption of high energy diets. Even then, TV viewing may not *cause* the type of diet consumed by the viewer, although Weicha's study suggests otherwise. Perhaps it is wise to agree with a common conclusion among epidemiologists that causal pathways are 'complex and interrelated' (Wake et al., 2003).

Misplaced worries about childhood obesity and digital technologies?

In our opinion concern about the rise in childhood *obesity* is not misplaced, given the links of weight gain in early life to lifelong health problems. Even if obese children do not grow into obese adults, a child of 10 years who develops weight-related diabetes or heart disease carries that burden for the remainder of their life. It is for this reason that some epidemiologists predict a shortened lifespan for the current generation of children. Our argument is that the media frame the problem too narrowly, risking exacerbating stigma and associated mental health problems and social distress: overweight and obese children are known to be at greater risk of depression than other children.

Since its introduction, television, a precursor to digital technologies, has been viewed with suspicion by numerous elites, including social scientists, anti-capitalist social movements and higher socioeconomic status groups. In one of the earliest studies of the impact of TV on social and family life, upper socioeconomic groups in the United States were found to have relatively low levels of TV ownership because they were 'concerned about the effects of TV on family life and school work, and in general disapprove of TV' (Maccoby, 1951, p. 422). Sociologists viewed it as transforming the impact of mass communications by exacerbating a sense of transience, and hence of 'timeliness, superficiality, and sensationalism in content' (Wright, 1975, p. 7). A former public relations and advertising executive famously wrote *Four Arguments for the Elimination of Television* (Mander, 1978). Apocalyptic and utopian scenarios about television's role in society are commonplace: Raymond Williams famously suggested that television, and associated technologies, would have inevitable, far-reaching consequences for cultural life in industrial nations, and predicted that 'The struggle over [how television is used] will reach into every corner of society' (Williams, 1974, p. 151).

In the field of obesity research, television's role as an alternative source of information and opinion to parents goes largely unremarked and under-investigated, beyond the influence of TV advertising. However, TV and DVDs provide a plethora of vivid perspectives on bodies: those that are 'normal', 'successful', 'unpopular', and so on. Much loved programs such as 'Home and Away', 'Neighbours', 'Big Brother' and 'The Biggest Loser' provide entrée to a world of bodily distinctions that parents find difficult to regulate and counter. Thus, not only does the digital age represent and fuel a generational divide where children are experts, it gives young people access to alternative sources of information and fantasy. In this way, digital technologies become an easy target for moral concern, and a potential source of multiple sins: sloth, gluttony, greed and envy.

While TV is heavily implicated as a risk factor for declines in physical activity, there are potentially stronger arguments to be made about other causes. Consistent documentation shows that there have been reductions in: children's participation in traditional team sports (Dollman et al., 2005); children's access to active physical education classes in schools (Salmon, Timperio, Cleland, & Venn, 2005); trips made wholly or partly by foot or cycle (Salmon, Timperio, Cleland, & Venn, 2005); and the amount of unsupervised discretionary or free time because of increasing hours spent in childcare and at school (Dollman et al., 2005).

While the evidence is mixed about the car's role in reducing children's physical activity levels (Dollman et al., 2005; Harten & Olds, 2004), the chapter by Hinde (this volume) makes a solid case for implicating this particular technology in rising levels of obesity for both adults and children. She points to a complex web of causation. Like television, the car shapes everyday life in the most fundamental and enduring ways. Roads carve up suburbs, making some parts inaccessible and other parts hard to penetrate, thereby constricting the space through which people can move on foot or bike. Like television and the Internet, cars provide viewing and auditory platforms for advertisements and other enticements for food and for passive play and entertainment opportunities. Each hour spent in the car displaces opportunities for active transport. However, only in rare exceptions (such as Ralph Nader's *Unsafe at Any Speed*) has the car attracted the opprobrium of television. There are, in short, numerous reasons to be wary of the fixation on digital technology in relation to population weight gain.

Place, socioeconomic status and children's weight

In contrast to the difficulties researchers have encountered connecting obesity and overweight to any singular determinant of physical activity, the linkages between socioeconomic status and unhealthy weight are well established (see the Friel and Broom chapter). In economically developed countries, children and adolescents from low income households are almost 1.5 times more likely to be overweight or obese than children from higher income households (Australian Institute of Health and Welfare,

2005; Lobstein et al., 2004; World Health Organization, 2000). If there is to be concern about children's weight then the inequalities in opportunities to enjoy normal weight, and its antecedents of at least moderate physical activity and a good diet, are arguably the major issues.

A Melbourne study of trends in physical activity between 1985 and 2001, a period when overweight and obesity doubled, found declines in the frequency of walking or cycling to school and the frequency of physical education (PE) lessons in school time, but not the frequency of school sport. Cycling and PE declined more in lower socioeconomic status areas, as did the rise in overweight and obesity (Salmon, Timperio, Cleland, & Venn, 2005). The researchers involved in this study expressed particular concern for the low levels of PE in low SES area schools, and they proposed a number of reasons for this finding: poorer resourcing of such schools, a lack of specialist PE teachers, difficulties attracting suitably skilled teachers, lack of commitment to PE, and pressure from parents to concentrate on more academic aspects of the curriculum.

Excessive television viewing also appears to have a social inequality dimension. It is a particular issue for children of women with fewer years of education, for children living in single-parent families and possibly for children of depressed mothers (Certain & Kahn, 2002; Gordon-Larsen et al., 2000; Lumeng et al., 2006; Salmon, Timperio, Cleland, & Venn, 2005). Such associations are of concern when the two-year-old toddlers of poorer and less educated women who watch more than the recommended two hours maximum of TV a day go on to become higher than recommended TV viewers at age six (Certain & Kahn, 2002). However, once again the causal chain is difficult to unravel with one study implicating a range of factors for excessive TV viewing and a different range of factors for low levels of physical activity, drawing the conclusion that TV viewing and low level activity are distinctive behaviours (Salmon, Timperio, Telford, Carver, & Crawford, 2005). Further, it appears that not all screen-based activities are socioeconomically determined: while television viewing and parental SES showed a relationship in the South Australian study, there was no such relationship with computer use or video game playing (Olds et al. 2006, p. 141).

Far from believing that children's excessive screen-based activities are a sign of poor parenting, we would argue that TV viewing is a symptom of a host of socioeconomic factors, including a lack of financial capacity to provide alternative pastimes. As the chapter by Banwell and colleagues indicates, television is a cheap activity compared with many others. Its appeal is magnified for those households characterised by low disposable income and lack of backyard space. Smaller backyards reduce the amount of free play, which is the most energy demanding for children.

There is also consistent corroboration that the quality of the neighbourhood is as important for some families as are their personal circumstances (Gordon-Larsen et al., 2000; Kavanagh et al., 2005). The neighbourhood structure affects active transport in a range of ways: the presence of major arterial roads, poor lighting, and agglomeration of neighbourhood shops into shopping centres all dampen physical activity (Olds et al., 2004, p. xviii). Perception of neighbourhood safety (Burdette & Whitaker, 2005) and high neighbourhood serious crime levels (Gordon-Larsen et al., 2000) are understandable determinants of children's activity levels, affecting the time spent in front of TV.

What is clear is that for most children, physical activity remains a popular pastime; however, their opportunities to choose to be active have been eroded over the years due to changes in a range of factors: in school policies; parenting styles; and rising parental concern about their children's safety, particularly in disadvantaged areas (Dollman et al., 2005). 'Asked what would help them to participate in sport, the most common responses from children were 'the ability to play with friends and family, and various logistical issues, such as transport, facilities and cost' (Olds et al. 2004, p. xvi). Clearly if mothers are worried about the safety of their neighbourhood, do not have a car or sufficient disposable income to spend on outings and sporting activities, and live in an area where the school does not invest in PE, then their children's range of options to be physically active are highly constrained. It is this constellation of circumstances that we believe needs discussing.

Why fixate on the activities of young people?

There are some good reasons, beyond potential health outcomes, for worrying about young people's leisure pursuits and use of technology. Children and young people are perhaps more intensively involved than adults in negotiating their sense of inclusion and belonging, or not. Through fashion and style, behaviour and play, publicly hanging out in groups and their favoured leisure activities they express their sense of belonging to particular sub-communities as well as to the wider community in which they live and go to school (Butcher & Thomas, 2003). A sense of belonging is created through the body, through embodied practices, by making bodies and their differences meaningful. Like adults, children and young people draw on diverse cultural resources to interpret their bodies and those of others, and to give expression to their belongingness, their sociality (Butcher & Thomas, 2003).

The body is culturally created, and this occurs under conditions of surveillance and of disciplinary regimes (Foucault, 1977; Foucault, 1984). Normative body types fluctuate and become dominant at specific historical times and places. Fat bodies are now disruptive in Western culture. They are viewed as causing trouble, as in need of greater surveillance and more intensive discipline. They are subject to assertions that they lack the will, the self-authorship, the power to locate themselves within the newly emerging community morality of self-regulated energy balance.

The question for public health policy makers thus becomes not merely promoting a message of controlling the food we eat and increasing activity levels. Rather, the question that needs to be addressed is how environments for meeting peers, displaying belonging and having fun together can become spaces of activity and inclusion, where all young people, including fat kids, can express their identities and affirm their sense of belonging alongside their peers. Taking an Aristotelian approach, the noted sports sociologist Norbet Elias argued for a conception of leisure as activity rather than as rest and relaxation (Elias & Dunning,

As the chapter by Denniss notes, it is the latter position that ng encouraged in adults at least. Furthermore, children will e encouraged to be active when family and neighbourhood circumstances are free of the types of constraints described in the previous section. Appeals to greater surveillance by authorities, including parents, may not be the best solution if children and young people can themselves be empowered to engage actively with public spaces displaying the physicality of their bodies, whatever their shape, to take pleasure in the spectacle, the diversity, the affirmation of belonging and bodily pleasure.

Conclusion

From a sociological perspective, an emphasis on the changing environment of children and young people as the cause of rising obesity rates is commendable. However, in targeting obesity or overweight for public health intervention, care must be taken to avoid adding to the stigmatisation and marginalisation of overweight and obese children and young people.

We do not argue that there is no reason for concern about weight among Australian youth; nor are we suggesting that use of digital technology for recreation is irrelevant to their rising rates of overweight and obesity. However, we do propose that the intensive focus on young people's activities (and lack of activity) represents several displacements which may have the effect of overemphasising one potentially comparatively minor piece of the puzzle, thus distracting attention from the wider range of factors that require attention (for example, car reliance). Indeed, blaming young people or their parents and their behaviour may have unintended and potentially deleterious effects on the very problem it is intended to address.

Implicit in the current media fixation are displacements:

- from adults (whose rates of unhealthy weight are unambiguously alarming) to children (where the evidence is more qualified);
- from those supposed to be responsible for their own choices to those thought to be more vulnerable to 'peer pressure'; and
- from people whose behaviour may be represented as firmly

established, onto those whose patterns might still be reshaped in more healthy directions.

The focus on any single technological determinant of overweight and obesity is similarly flawed, ushering in further displacements: particularly from public and political responsibility for making physical and social habitats conducive to physical activity and bodily expressions, onto parental and individual responsibility to regulate behaviours. Together, these displacements express traditional anxieties about the young, and deflect attention from the responsibility of adults for their own weight-related problems and, perhaps more significantly, from the responsibility of social institutions to create environments conducive to health (including healthy weight) for young and old alike.

SIN#5:
THE CAR-RELIANT
ENVIRONMENT

The vehicle that drives obesity

Sarah Hinde

ustralia's obsession with the car is rarely characterised as sinful. More often, the automobile is cast as a superior form of mobility, conferring freedom and status to those who use it. For some decades, public health has been alerting us to the health dangers of modern car worship including high rates of injury and death on the roads, the detrimental effects of exposure to air pollution and noise, and longer term concerns such as the major contribution of road transport to greenhouse gas emissions. Researchers are now implicating the car in rising rates of obesity. Some studies have shown a statistical relationship between car transport and risk of obesity for individuals. The question remains, however, what is the role of the automobile in rising obesity rates?

The car is essential to the structure of today's society, the workings of the economy and even the way people go about their everyday routines. It enables people to live a busy, harried life, yet remain sedentary and isolated from one another. Motor vehicles facilitate the rapid movement of workers, goods and consumers across space; indeed, the automobile is a major item of mass production and consumption, a significant commodity that helped kick off this era of materialism. The car underpinned suburbanisation and facilitated the spatial consolidation of retail centres for provisioning of food, other commodities and entertainment. This spatial transformation rendered the car essential for social participation, and displaced other forms of mobility such as walking, cycling and public transport. The automobile permeates all aspects of Australian society: as a form of mobility, an economic object, geographic determinant and cultural icon. In so doing, the automobile should not be seen as just a common sedentary pastime, but as a powerful 'vehicle' for many social trends that together render Australia's environment obesogenic.

The problem of Australia's car reliance

It is widely acknowledged that Australia's transport systems are dominated by the automobile (Mees 2000; Laird et al. 2001). Among the 20-odd million people in Australia, around 12 million are licensed to drive with about 12 million registered vehicles that enable them to do so (Hinde & Dixon, 2005). Figure 1 illustrates how the vast majority of Australian households have access to at least one motor vehicle. In fact, almost half of Australian households have at least two motor vehicles (Australian Bureau of Statistics, 2002).

FIGURE 1 Australian households with and without access to a motor vehicle (Australian Bureau of Statistics, 2002)

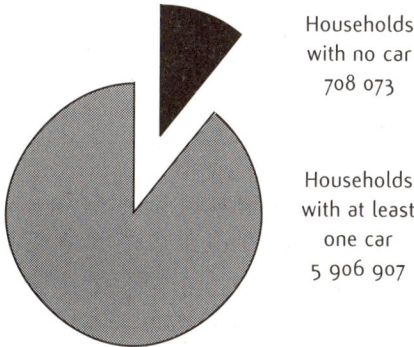

Households
with no car
708 073

Households
with at least
one car
5 906 907

But a car-reliant nation doesn't just own lots of cars: Australia supports the use of the motor vehicle to the point that life without it would be 'unimaginable' (Hinde & Dixon, 2005). This country offers, for example, generous road provision, and some of the cheapest petrol in the developed world (Austroads, 2000). In such an environment that fosters the use of the automobile, it is unsurprising that Australian cities rank among the most 'car dependent' cities in the world (Laird et al., 2001).

The motor vehicle performs the majority of the transport tasks of getting people to and from their workplace. For almost all Australians travelling to work every day, only one mode of transport is used and these have been represented in figure 2. This graph shows how more than four in every five people travelling to work use a motor vehicle; the motor vehicle share vastly outweighs the total contribution made by public transport, walking, cycling and other modes (for example, motorbikes and scooters). Of those Australians who use a car, most drive themselves. So, 75 per cent of Australian workers drive to their workplace and a further 8 per cent get there as car passengers (ABS, 2002).

FIGURE 2 Modes of transport used by Australians to get to work (Australian Bureau of Statistics, 2002)

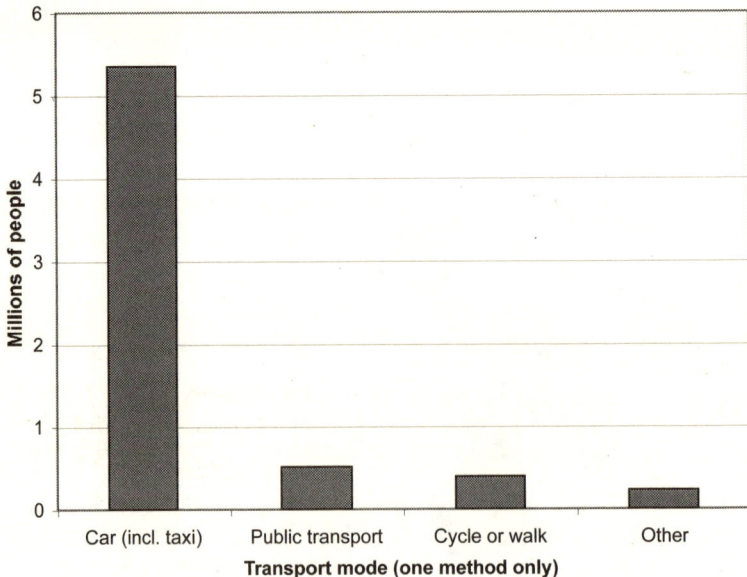

Adults are not the only heavy users of car transport. Children are increasingly being chauffeured to school rather than travelling by foot or bicycle. A survey of over 1000 families from 19 Melbourne primary schools revealed that less than half of 5 and 6 year olds, and less than two-thirds of 10–12 year olds, walk or cycle to school once a week or more (Timperio et al., 2004).

The collective distance travelled by Australians each year has inter-planetary dimensions! The ABS reported that in a 12-month period, Australia's vehicles had together travelled 'the equivalent of going to Pluto and back 23 times' (ABS, 2003). Australians are spending growing quantities of time accelerating across ever-increasing distances. The total kilometres travelled in Australia grew 80 per cent in the 20 years to 1998; this rate of growth was more than double population growth for the period (Austroads, 2000).

The numerous sustainability concerns relating to our heavy car reliance have been highlighted for decades. More recently, there has been a growing acknowledgment of the detrimental effects of the automobile on the population's health. The World Health Organization (WHO) delivered a comprehensive and accessible review of the various known population health impacts of transport around the globe (Dora & Phillips 2000), and Australian researchers have begun to alert us to these consequences in Australia (McMichael, 2001; Mason, 2000a; Mason, 2000b; Kjellstrom et al., 2003). The major known detrimental consequences are summarised in box 1.

Research into the plethora of damaging health consequences together suggests that the continued dominance of the motor vehicle is having massive negative results for the world's population, now and into the future. Car reliance appears to be unsustainable, demanding huge resources and causing environmental damage, inequities in mobility and ill-health effects. Environmentalists, epidemiologists, urban planners, geographers, sociologists and more recently public health researchers, governments and international bodies have declared the need for our societies to move away from car reliance.

BOX 1

Apart from the multiple influences of car reliance on physical activity and food consumption, there are many other significant negative impacts on the health and wellbeing of our community:

Oil vulnerability ... Production of oil will peak, and some research suggests it probably already has. Within our lifetimes, we will begin to feel the impact of running out of oil. This won't just change the modes and costs of getting around but will shape the very nature of transport, and Australia's economy and culture which currently depends so heavily on the motor vehicle.

Congestion ... This is another issue that challenges the sustainability of a car-reliant transport system. Individualised, motorised technology takes up an inordinate amount of room when compared to more space efficient modes such as buses, trams and especially trains. The upshot is that our cities must convert more and more surfaces to asphalt. NSW Sustainability Commissioner Peter Newman (2005) provides a stark illustration using the Australian landmark sports stadium, the Melbourne Cricket Ground (MCG): 'the 200,000 people a day coming into Sydney by train would need 65 freeway lanes and ... [the] equivalent to 520 carparks the size of the MCG' if they were to use a car instead.

Motor vehicle accidents causing disability and death ... This is the leading cause of death for males aged 15–24; and traffic crashes account for half of the health impact of injury, being the principal cause of death for people under 45 years (Mathers et al., 1999).

Pollution ... Small particles, carbon monoxide, ozone, benzene and lead are some of the pollutants arising from the automobile; these have been linked to respiratory disease and other respiratory symptoms including asthma, cardiovascular disease and cancer (Dora & Phillips, 2000).

Major contribution to greenhouse gas emissions and therefore climate change ... The impact of climate change, such as increased frequency of extreme weather events and changes in the ecology of disease vectors (for example, mosquitoes), may have potentially disastrous health consequences (McMichael, 2001).

Noise disturbance ... The noise generated on roads and

freeways has been linked to problems such as impaired communication, disturbed sleep, difficulties with performance, annoyance, increased aggression, heart disease and hypertension, and hearing impairment (Dora & Phillips, 2000).

Community disruption ... Roads and freeways cause major disruption to spaces where people live. The car's ongoing dominance demands that green spaces and other places where social life occurs be destroyed and replaced with non-human places like roads and car parks. Roads also divide communities: politically, as the costs and benefits of roads are attributed to different segments of the community; and physically, by imposing structures and causing major impediments to human movement between different parts of the city. Moreover, Australian transport researcher Paul Mees (2000) points out how the imperatives of a car-based transport system tend to thwart the development of alternative forms of mobility, leading to increasing inequities in mobility and therefore access to society's resources (Mees, 2000).

Car use and obesity risk

Australian obesity experts, coming from a range of sectors and disciplines, acknowledge the social importance of car reliance in Australia's obesity epidemic. Australian researchers interviewed 50 food and physical activity experts about the social trends contributing to the rise in obesity rates in this country, and car reliance was named by many of them. In a subsequent ranking exercise, car reliance was most frequently ranked as the 'most important' trend leading to declines in physical activity, and had the highest average 'importance' rank across all the social trends named (Banwell, Hinde et al., 2005).

In the first major published study of travel and weight, American researchers provided individual-level survey evidence that daily time spent in the motor vehicle is correlated with risk of being overweight or obese (Frank et al., 2004). Their survey of over 10 000 people in the United States showed that for every 60 minutes spent in the motor vehicle, the probability of a person being obese increases by 6 per cent. This relationship between car travel and obesity occurred over and above the effects of urban environment and other variables such as socioeconomic status and age. Disturbingly, time spent in the car ranged up to more than five hours per day for a small number of the more disadvantaged participants, translating to a 30 per cent increase in risk of obesity for those people.

A relationship between driving and risk of overweight and obesity has recently been demonstrated in New South Wales. A survey of almost 7000 people showed that those who drive a car to work were 13 per cent more likely to be overweight or obese than those who do not. Car drivers were also less likely to achieve adequate levels of physical activity each day (Wen et al., 2006).

In other, smaller studies focusing on children there has been mixed evidence about the relationship between car transport and weight. For example, a small United States study of 320 children suggested active commuting on its own does not affect body mass index (BMI) in children (Heelan et al., 2005), however a larger survey of 1518 Filipino children indicated that travelling to school in a car probably contributed a weight gain of around 1 kilogram per year (Tudor-Locke et al., 2003).

These studies offer little guidance on the specific mechanisms that may be causing car transport to increase obesity risk. The most common hypothesis is that physical activity is displaced when people use a motor vehicle instead of an 'active transport' mode such as walking, cycling or using public transport (Mason, 2000a; Mason, 2000b). It is argued the habit-forming potential of the automobile consolidates this displacement of physical activity, as the car becomes the default or automatic mode of transport, even when active transport might be feasible, convenient and even preferred (Handy et al., 2005).

This widespread assumption about displacement of physical activity is backed by some research evidence that confirms and quantifies this relationship. For example, one study of 10–13-year-old children in the United Kingdom showed that walking for transport offers the greatest quantity of high intensity activity for children (Mackett et al., 2005). While physical education classes at school offered slightly more intense exercise, these contributed fewer hours of activity across the week, rendering walking for transport the overall greatest source of exercise in children (Mackett et al., 2005).

While it seems likely that displacement of active transport by the motor vehicle contributes to obesity risk, much research suggests that levels of physical activity are shaped by multiple factors. For example, a recent large survey of over 2000 Melbourne residents highlighted the importance of geographical and social context in determining whether people were physically active, including whether they walked or cycled for transport (Kavanagh et al., 2005). These researchers emphasised the importance of such factors as local facilities, urban form, safety and the extent of neighbourhood socioeconomic deprivation in shaping the activity levels of residents.

Other research has shown that socioeconomically deprived people are often compelled to use so-called 'active transport' but that this is severely detrimental to their health (Bostock, 2001). This research described the stressful experience of deprived people who have no alternative to walking for transport: they are compelled to walk long distances, through unsafe neighbourhoods, along dangerous roads, carrying heavy bags and often while supervising small, tired children.

This mixed evidence about cars, physical activity, wellbeing and weight together suggests that the relationships are more complex than they may first seem. The health impacts of car reliance must depend on the social, economic and geographic context in which the car, or other, transport takes place. In an effort to move beyond the commonly presumed 'habitual laziness' hypothesis, other possible mechanisms are listed in box 2. The remainder of this chapter is concerned with the broader social role of the motor vehicle and the specific implications for rising rates of obesity.

The road to obesity

The automobile is a literal and metaphorical 'vehicle' for many of the obesity-promoting social changes of the last century. The marks of automobility can be observed from multiple perspectives:

in our urban environments, the economy, and as part of people's everyday routines. Above and beyond its sedentary nature, the car's contribution to obesity permeates multiple obesogenic trends. This section describes how car reliance is both obesogenic in its own right and has been instrumental to many of the other social trends that are described in more detail throughout this book.

BOX 2

Most Australian workers use a motor vehicle to get to work every day, and this is also the main form of transport used for other daily activities like getting the kids to school and doing the shopping. It isn't just the habitual displacement of active transport that might be contributing to rising rates of obesity:

A place to eat ... Most people travel alone in their vehicle and the car offers them a private, uninhibited environment. People look forward to their time in the car as recreation, and an opportunity to sing to the radio at the top of their voices. The lack of social inhibition in the car provides the perfect setting for the 'gastro-anomie' (Fischler, 1988) of the modern world whereby structured, convivial mealtimes are replaced by solitary, unstructured grazing on food and drinks. Mindless grazing can while away the minutes and hours on long trips along anonymous freeways or time-consuming waits in peak-hour traffic; and strategic food treats for the kids can distract them from the eternal question of 'when are we going to get there?'.

The 'motorised shopping trolley' ... The automobile is not just a setting for food consumption; it is the major tool for obtaining food (Hinde & Dixon, 2005). The car enhances access to food, especially from outlets that cater especially to vehicle users such as 'drive-thru' fast-food outlets and service stations that offer snacks and drinks as well as petrol. Perhaps more significantly, the capacity to shift large volumes of food in the boot means it is the primary tool in food provisioning. The car enables people to shop at large, centralised supermarkets for their weekly, or even fortnightly, provisions. This shift from locally sourced, pedestrian shopping to car-based supermarket shopping enhances access to a range of mass-produced and pre-prepared products that increase intake of energy from foods.

Road rage ... The experience of driving itself may have implications for subsequent eating and physical inactivity. For example, some women state they find driving stressful and would prefer not to use the car if it were possible (Dowling, 2000). Congestion and noise are thought to contribute to mental health problems, child development issues and stress levels (Dora & Phillips, 2000). Australia stands out in the world as having among the highest levels of 'road rage' with one in ten people experiencing a physical attack or threat of physical attack in the last 12 months (Drugs and Crime Prevention Committee, 2005). Such high levels of car-related stress may, for example, lead people to emotional overeating or to seek out sedentary, introverted leisure activities for stress relief.

A captive audience ... Car drivers and passengers are also exposed to a range of advertising media including roadside billboards, radio advertising and shopfront signage, and increasingly, via televisions built into cars. Increasing attention is being paid to the role of television advertising in childhood obesity. Children are spending more time as car passengers being chauffeured to school and extracurricular activities (ironically, so they will be safe from traffic). Their exposure to advertising during travel time may be just as potent as television advertising at home.

Shaping the physical environment

The automobile has fundamentally shaped the way modern cities are designed; and the car has become an unnoticed and almost invisible part of the cityscape. As automobiles became popular in Australia during the middle of the last century, residents were no longer constrained to the rail networks in locating their housing. Roads extended in all directions and houses were built in turn; this phenomenon is called urban sprawl (ABS, 2001). Car reliance has also facilitated the dispersal of daily activities beyond the local neighbourhood, including schooling, industrial and commercial sites (that is, workplaces) and leisure. These changes have also brought with them car-only environments such as freeways, tunnels, 'drive-in' and 'drive-thru' (Beckmann, 2001). The car is therefore a primary constituent of people's physical surroundings.

A landscape that is dominated by the automobile is generally not conducive to alternative forms of mobility such as walking, cycling and public transport (Mees, 2000). Studies looking into 'walkability' of areas have shown that an overwhelming presence of car traffic reduces people's inclination to walk in the area. Decision to walk depends on functional, safety, aesthetic and destination aspects of the trip and a car-dominated environment is more likely to have poor safety, many crossings, pollution and less visual appeal (Pikora et al., 2003). Furthermore, a city that is built with the car in mind is more likely to have destinations that are relatively inaccessible to pedestrians. For example, destinations are too far away to walk, can only be reached via a convoluted route, or are impeded or made more dangerous by major roadways.

Child pedestrians respond differently to the urban form than adult pedestrians. For example, adults are more likely to walk in a neighbourhood with many street intersections, but this 'connectivity' seems to reduce the likelihood of walking for children. Australian research highlights the importance of such environmental factors that deter parents from letting their child walk or cycle; for example, heavy traffic, few crossings, steep hills, and the perception of few other children walking or cycling in the neighbourhood (Timperio, Crawford et al., 2004; Timperio, Bell et al., 2006).

Heightened parental concern about traffic safety (and changes in parenting more generally, discussed in the chapter by Banwell and colleagues) has led to parents introducing more structure into children's lives. As illustrated in figure 3, a vicious cycle has emerged, whereby concerns about child pedestrian safety have compelled parents to chauffeur their children to school, which in turn increases traffic and parent worry. Growing traffic has also inspired the replacement of unstructured play with the following:

- structured and organised sports, which offer less overall physical activity than would active transport or unstructured play; also, when these activities are reached by car, instead of walking, less exercise intensity is obtained (Mackett et al., 2005);
- other extracurricular activities that are not physically demanding; and
- leisure time at home, which is also regarded as less physically active than any activity away from the home (Mackett et al., 2005), perhaps reflecting the increasing sedentarisation of leisure activities (the topic of another chapter).

FIGURE 3 How car reliance is changing children's physical activity (from Hinde & Dixon, 2005)

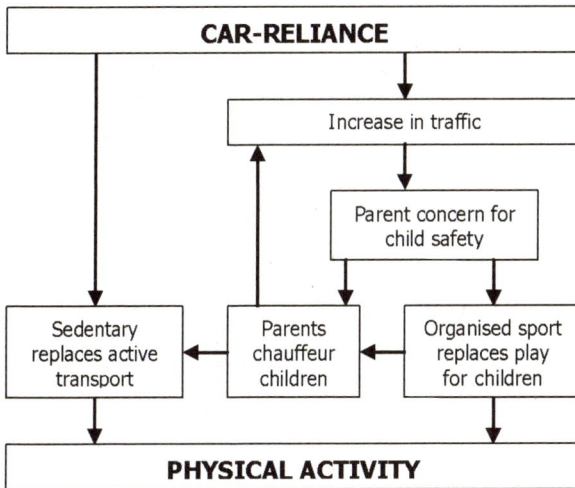

The car-centred urban form has also changed people's practices in purchasing and consuming food (Banwell, Dixon et al., 2005). Suburbanisation has allowed the agglomeration and centralisation of shops into malls and retail districts (Beckmann, 2001). Australians mostly purchase their food from large supermarkets as opposed to, say, the 'Mediterranean' model of neighbourhood vendors supplying regional produce and locally made items. Supermarket food shopping is more sedentary and the nature of the food purchased is more likely to be mass produced and/or pre-prepared, delivering more calories. Car-dependent shopping malls have other implications for obesity rates too, facilitating a range of sedentary leisure: cinema, equipment-intensive computer games, attendance at 'food courts' that offer a suite of fast-food options, not to mention 'shopping' itself – the sedentary pastime of the ideal consumer.

AN ECONOMIC DRIVER

The automobile industry is peculiar because it has a dual economic function: it offers industry 'the capability to commodify means of mobility, and at the same time accelerate the movement of goods and people in the economy' (Paterson, 2000, p. 265). Cars and car-related goods are profitable commodities in their own right. Motor vehicles also serve the purpose of moving other commodities from sites of production to wholesale and retail outlets. Importantly, the automobile also equips workers and consumers to get to places where they work, buy goods and receive services. The movement of people and things is essential to the economy, and much of the economic cost of this movement is borne by the workers and consumers themselves (Paterson, 2000).

The car industry has also been instrumental in the increasing materialism of today's society (see the Denniss chapter). The auto sector is the home of 'Fordism': this industry was a leader in developing mass production techniques and shaping labour relations. It was therefore also instrumental in bringing about mass consumption, whereby mass production depended on a new 'regime of accumulation' that underpins the materialistic tendencies of modern society.

Mass consumption of the motor vehicle persists just as strongly today. Sales of new motor vehicles continue to rise, for passenger vehicles and especially sports utility vehicles (SUVs) – the latter are better known in Australia as four-wheel drives (4WDs). Figure 4 illustrates how monthly sales of both vehicle types have grown over the last ten years, the rate of growth being especially rapid for 4WDs. Passenger vehicle sales have grown from 38 000 vehicles per month in 1994 to over 50 000 per month in 2005; in addition, average monthly sales of 4WDs were 4000 in 1994 and had almost quadrupled to over 15 000 per month by 2005 (ABS, 2005).

The rapid growth of ownership of 4WDs relative to passenger vehicles means the market in new car sales is increasingly tipping in their favour. Table 1 presents the annual ratios of new passenger vehicle to 4WD monthly sales (ABS, 2005). In 1994 the ratio was more than 10:1 and now that ratio is getting closer to 3:1. That means that for every seven new passenger vehicles sold in 2005, two 4WDs were also purchased.

FIGURE 4 Trend in monthly sales of passenger and sports utility vehicles 1994—2005 (Australian Bureau of Statistics, 2005)

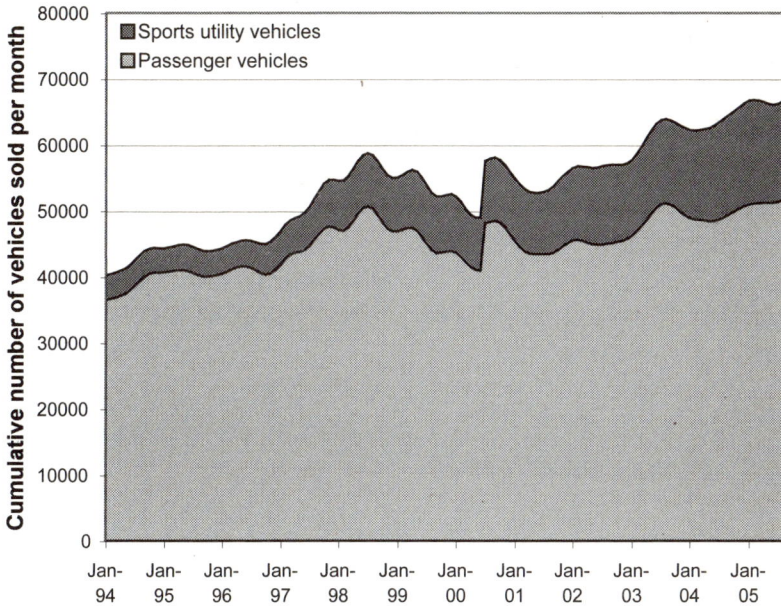

A recent survey reported by The Australia Institute (Hamilton & Barbato, 2005) illustrates how this shift towards 4WDs parallels many of the modern obesogenic trends discussed in this book. The report explained that although 4WD owners declare an enjoyment of physical activity, American market researchers find that people who buy 4WDs 'tend to like fine restaurants a lot more than off-road driving'. Indeed, these commentators suggest that marketing has played a key role in the growing popularity of 4WDs. The survey also showed that consumers of 4WDs generally have more individualistic attitudes and are less concerned about the community at large; they are more nervous about parenthood; and are doubly likely than the rest of the population to say 'I was born to shop'. Finally, the data indicated that 4WD owners are more likely to be obese (Hamilton & Barbato, 2005).

TABLE 1 Average annual ratios of passenger to sports utility vehicle (SUV) monthly sales 1994–2005 (Australian Bureau of Statistics, 2005)

Year	Ratio passenger vehicles: SUV sales
1994	10.22
1995	10.80
1996	9.88
1997	7.67
1998	6.09
1999	5.33
2000	5.25
2001	4.57
2002	3.92
2003	3.92
2004	3.42
2005 (to Sept)	3.34

AN EVERYDAY PART OF LIFE

Australian obesity experts believe that a lack of time, or sense of 'busyness' has been a major contributor to falling physical activity levels and changing food consumption patterns (Banwell, Hinde et al., 2005). Chapters by Broom and Strazdins, and Banwell and colleagues more fully explore this relationship; however, some obesity experts:

... thought that lack of time was a perception while others noted the pressure on people to do more with their time, related to a need to achieve success, to comply with work demands, and to be a good parent by setting aside time for children's activities ... Accompanying this is the sense that lives are more complicated and require sophisticated feats of organisation to be manageable ... Considerable social pressure forces people to use their time efficiently and to adopt modern conveniences to save time. (Banwell, Hinde' et al., 2005, p. 567)

The automobile is often thought to be the best solution to the pressing demands of daily life; however, it is likely that car reliance is also an underlying cause of this sense of 'busyness'. The effect of living our lives at venues that are distributed across great distances is that it increases the pace of life (Sheller & Urry, 2000). The demands of getting to and from various destinations become squeezed, and the car eventually becomes the only option for travelling. The freedom and autonomy originally offered by the car is therefore displaced by the necessity of having a car to survive the pace of life. The automobile 'make[s] complex, harried patterns of social life ... just about possible' (Sheller & Urry, 2000, p. 744). This cycle of expanding distances and the mounting pressure to fit many destinations into one day becomes more acute as congestion worsens, and the motor vehicle becomes its own worst enemy (Freund & Martin, 1996).

The car is promoted as the most efficient or convenient option, but in many cases it is actually the only option for meeting daily demands and participating in modern life; an invisible 'second-nature' (Miller, 2001). The motor car has transformed every aspect of our daily lives:

> ... the food we eat, the music we listen to, the risks we take, the places we visit, the errands we run, the emotions we feel, the movies we watch, the money we spend, the stress we endure and the air we breathe. (Wollen, 2002, p. 11)

The automobile is commonly regarded as critical to fulfilling one's maternal responsibilities. A qualitative study revealed that Australian women feel committed to owning a motor vehicle, because it equips them to most effectively manage their household responsibilities (Dowling, 2000). For example, in a single day, one

Sydney mother described driving her husband to and from work, and making separate trips to swimming, a mother's meeting and the shops. I have heard similar stories during interviews with mothers living in Melbourne, who daily travel to far-flung destinations to visit parents, parents-in-law, swimming lessons, playgroup, kinder gym, shopping malls, specialty shops in other suburbs, a plethora of health and medical appointments, organised sport and social activities.

Beyond the management of their daily tasks, the mothers interviewed by Dowling (2000) described how an automobile allows a parent to optimise the opportunities they provide for their children. For example, it allows a parent to choose among schools outside their local area, so they can find a school that will suit the particular needs or interests of the child. Here, the motor vehicle can be seen to be facilitating a general trend in child-focused parenting as well as reinforcing the division of household labour between the genders, which are both issues of concern when considering the obesogenic environment (see the chapter by Banwell and colleagues).

Mothers are not the only people reliant on an automobile – as this chapter has described, most Australians depend on car transport. Melbourne residents describe their use of the motorcar to ferry equipment required for work or sport, to escape the bustle of the city and go bushwalking on weekends, to do their grocery shopping at the markets or supermarket on the weekends, to get around when injury makes walking or catching public transport too difficult, to transport their pet dog to a 'dogs off leash' park for exercise, or to be on-call in case of an emergency. On closer inspection, it appears that the automobile has been sewn into the fabric of most Australians' everyday existence.

A FALSE GOD?

Car reliance is one of the few social causes of obesity not generally deemed 'sinful'. Rather, the car is often portrayed romantically, as in this history of the automobile in Australia:

> Like a human love affair, our love affair with the car unfolded, step by step, from its first moment of distant admiration

through casual acquaintance, infatuation and deep bonding to taken-for-granted familiarity. (Davison, 2004, p. xii)

However, planning and health researchers from the United States have pointed out: 'obesity, inactivity, depression, and loss of community have not "happened" to us. We legislated, subsidized, and planned it this way' (Frumkin et al., 2004). Car reliance has not been a story of natural human evolution but rather a history of human action, with vast social consequences.

Much legislation, subsidisation and planning has encouraged the uptake and use of the motor vehicle (Hinde & Dixon, 2005). For example, all three levels of government together spend $A23 million per working day on roads (Austroads, 2000). Weighing government revenue (for example, tax) against the various costs to the community of the current car-dominated transport system, Australian researchers suggest that the 'road deficit' amounted to $A19 billion per year prior to the introduction of the new tax system, which was expected to increase the net deficit in 2000–01 (Laird et al., 2001). This investment by government in turn permits the flourishing of industries such as steel, car manufacture, road building and construction; namely, some of the most powerful industries in the world. And shareholders are not the only ones who gain from the automobile's dominance; for example, one out of every ten jobs in the industrialised world is directly related to the car (Paterson, 2000).

The automobile hasn't just entrenched itself economically, it has also firmly fixed itself into the hearts and minds of Australians. The role of the car and related industries, and indeed the car itself as an object of mass consumption, played integral roles in the development of countries like America and Australia. The automobile came to be regarded as 'perhaps *the* symbol of progress for most of the last century' (Paterson, 2000). As such, when car sales hit new bumper levels, Australian Treasurer Peter Costello (Commonwealth Treasurer, 2004) describes how this is 'good' for everyone: 'the manufacturers … the people who are employed in the retail end of the car industry, and best of all it is good for consumers who have bought more cars than have ever been sold in Australia before'.

It takes more than just owning a vehicle to reap the benefits of automobility: the motorist depends on an entire system of use including roads, road rules, car parks and petrol stations (Beckmann, 2001; Freund & Martin, 1996). This system of use must be addressed when contemplating the relationship between transport and obesity. It isn't just the aforementioned 60 minutes sitting in the car that increases obesity risk by 6 per cent, but the system that necessitates those 60 minutes in the car, with all the social implications, that are the ultimate culprits; the 'sins' of the modern environment.

Conclusion

This chapter has elaborated on the ways in which Australia's reliance on the automobile is not good or virtuous but rather health damaging and obesity promoting. The entrenchment of the motor vehicle across all aspects of modern social life means it is implicated in many obesogenic social trends. The car has not only displaced alternative, healthier and more equitable forms of mobility; it has facilitated a system of values, industries and physical settings that promote consumption of high energy food and prevent physical activity. The road to wellbeing for all Australians demands that we interrogate our value systems, question our economic imperatives and pay attention to the design of our cities to ensure they all support and facilitate healthy ways of life.

SIN#6:
THE MARKETED ENVIRONMENT

Formula for fatness

*Julie Smith**

More than 25 years ago, epidemiological research showed links between formula feeding in infancy and higher incidence of overweight and obesity in adolescence, a connection originally proposed in the 1920s. Only recently, however, has there been sufficient methodologically robust research to confirm the relationship. It has also been found that mothers who do not breastfeed typically retain more weight after childbirth. Though less obvious than adult addictions to junk food and slothful lifestyles, poor infant feeding practices contribute to rising obesity in Australia.

Researchers focusing on adults or older children commonly assume that metabolism is fixed, so that weight gain results simply from eating too much and exercising too little. However, evidence is accumulating that artificial infant feeding during past

* I am grateful for helpful comments on drafts of this chapter from Annemarie Jutel, Louise Bartlett, Dorothy Broom, Jane Dixon and Mark Dunstone, and Maureen Minchin. Nancy Cinnadao collected the advertising data. Responsibility for the final paper and any remaining errors and omissions is entirely my own.

decades has altered people's metabolisms and eating behaviours, predisposing them to overweight or obesity in later life.

Just as anti-smoking campaigns focus on the smoker, the 'blame' for premature weaning from breastfeeding easily falls onto mothers. Mothers commonly report feeling guilty about not breastfeeding. The Commonwealth Health Minister Tony Abbott was recently reported as saying on obesity that 'the only person responsible for what goes into my mouth is me, and the only people who are responsible for what goes into kids' mouths are the parents' (*Sydney Morning Herald*, 12 April 2006, p. 4).

As mammals, mothers are biologically designed to breastfeed, but from the 1950s in Australia, many did not. There was a sharp decline in breastfeeding, and rapid growth in the mass market for commercial artificial infant feeding products. This move away from breastfeeding is an element of the current obesity problem. It has come about due to an alliance of industry and medicine in marketing commercial artificial infant feeding products since the 1950s.

Thus the 'mass mammary malfunction' evident from the 1950s was not due to the 'sins of the mothers' (now being visited on future generations as an obesity problem), but the result of supposedly 'scientific' beliefs and health institutional practices which helped create and expand the market for new commercial infant feeding products.

Obesity and infant nutrition

PUBLIC POLICY FRAMEWORK: BREASTFEEDING AND OBESITY

In 2003 Australia's National Obesity Task Force reported that about 1.5 million Australians under 18 were overweight or obese. The proportion of children who were overweight tripled between 1985 and 1995 and continues to rise. The Task Force noted that 'effective prevention needs responses from all parts of society to encourage more active living and healthy living, beginning from the very start of life with breastfeeding' (Commonwealth of Australia, 2003, p. 3). It listed 'breastfeeding' as a 'setting' that was a key 'best-buy' government response to the problem of obesity.

The same year, the World Health Organization (WHO) Expert

Report on *Diet, Nutrition and the Prevention of Chronic Diseases* (2003) also cited inadequate breastfeeding as a possible risk factor for chronic disease. It found 'increasingly strong evidence that a lower risk of developing obesity may be directly related to the length of exclusive breastfeeding although it may not become evident until later in childhood' (p. 32). Since then several studies and reviews have identified artificial feeding in infancy as a significant risk factor for key components of the 'metabolic syndrome' – overweight, high blood pressure and cholesterol, heart disease and diabetes (American Academy of Pediatrics, 2005).

Recognising that overfeeding is as much malnutrition as underfeeding, and that breastfed infants represent the biological norm, the WHO has recently developed revised indicators and new weight charts based on exclusively breastfed infants (World Health Organization, 2006). Previous charts overestimated infant energy needs, and resulted in overfeeding, excessive weight gain and premature weaning of infants from breastmilk.

WHO recommendations for optimal infant feeding are for exclusive breastfeeding to 6 months with continued breastfeeding (along with appropriate complementary foods) to 2 years and beyond (World Health Assembly [Fifty Fourth] 2001). This is reflected in Australia's *Dietary Guidelines for Children*, though still not yet implemented in food standards and labelling requirements, government sponsored infant advisory services or health professional codes of conduct.

Recognising the important role of maternity care services in establishing breastfeeding, WHO and UNICEF have developed ten evidence-based 'steps' to successful breastfeeding (WHO Division of Child Health and Development, 1998). There is growing evidence that large improvements in exclusive breastfeeding rates can be achieved at the population level (Kramer et al., 2002; Quinn et al., 2005). Central to reducing early weaning is abandoning hospital policies and practices that, as we shall see, have been widespread for several decades since introduced in the 1930s.

INFANT NUTRITION AND OBESITY: THE LINKS

Until recently, studies were unclear on the relationship between infant nutrition and later obesity because of weaknesses in research design. The widespread use of cows milk for infant feeding up to the 1970s, the changing contents of infant formula and the varied diets of mothers also makes it difficult to draw conclusive evidence on the effect of artificial feeding. However, a systematic review of several new large and well-designed studies in the early 1990s (Dewey, 2003) found that non-breastfed infants were 30–50 per cent more likely to be overweight in childhood and adolescence than breastfed infants, though there remained the possibility that factors such as parental attributes and family environment had not been fully accounted for.

More recent systematic reviews and meta-analyses have also found that artificial infant feeding increases the likelihood of childhood obesity. For example, a meta-analysis of nine studies of around 69 000 participants found the odds of childhood obesity were 28 per cent higher among formula fed infants (pooled adjusted odds ratio 0.78) (Arenz et al., 2004). A 2005 review of 28 studies with 298 900 participants (Owen et al., 2005) concluded that not having been breastfed increased the risk of later obesity by 15 per cent compared to those who were breastfed; the effects were even stronger where breastfeeding was exclusive or more prolonged.

Researchers have also found that the shorter the duration of breastfeeding, the greater the likelihood of later obesity. A meta-analysis examining 17 different studies with around 121 000 participants found that the longer the duration of breastfeeding, the lower the risk of childhood overweight/obesity (Harder et al., 2005). The risk of overweight/obesity was reduced by 4 per cent for each month of breastfeeding, with a 9 month duration reducing risk by over 30 per cent compared to breastfeeding for less than a month. Such a dose-responsive relationship suggests causation, making it implausible that an association is due to confounding factors. Another recent study of 2500 siblings showed that those breastfed for a longer duration (four months on average) had a 6–8 per cent lower chance of being overweight in adolescence (Gillman et al., 2006). This study suggests that apparently protective effects of breastfeeding are not due to unmeasured sociocultural factors because the association of breastfeeding duration with adolescent obesity for siblings raised in the same family environment was similar to the results for the whole sample.

Although the magnitude of the effect of artificial infant feeding on later obesity is moderate, it is likely to be of public health importance because so few infants are optimally breastfed and obesity is affecting such a large proportion of the population. It has been estimated that the population attributable risk of overweight from formula feeding in the United States is between 15 and 20 per cent (Dietz, 2001). Increasing the initiation rate and duration of breastfeeding has the potential to significantly reduce the long-term risk of becoming overweight or obese compared to other primary and secondary health interventions, many of which are expensive and do not have such lasting effects over the long term (Plagemann & Harder, 2005).

HOW FEEDING IN INFANCY AFFECTS LATER RISK OF OBESITY

The mechanisms by which breastfeeding reduces obesity risk are still unclear, but are probably through the metabolic programming effects of human milk, as well as from effects on infant and maternal feeding behaviour.

Breastfeeding facilitates development of self-control, and may also shape later food preferences towards healthy eating, as components of human milk and the suckling experience affect feeding behaviours of the mother and the child.

- Although infants can self-regulate energy intake, artificially fed infants have less self-control over how much milk they will take (Birch & Fisher, 1998). Partly this is because the carer has more control over the formula fed infant's intake and may keep feeding even when the baby is full (Fomon et al., 1975). It may also relate to more vigorous feeding (larger feeds and higher sucking pressure) associated with bottle feeding (Agras et al., 1987; Lucas et al., 1979).

- Parental interference, such as encouragement to eat or excessive food restrictions, can override the development of self-control in children and increase obesity risk (Ventura et al., 2005). Studies show that as breastfeeding mothers cannot easily monitor and manipulate milk intake, their feeding style is more responsive to infant feeding cues of hunger and satiety (Taveras et al., 2004). Reinforcing this is the common view that a heavy infant is a sign of successful feeding and parenting (Baughcum et al., 1998).

- As the taste of breastmilk varies with the mother's diet, breastfed babies accept new foods more readily (Sullivan & Birch, 1994). This is significant because infants naturally resist eating new foods and prefer sweet or salty tastes (Birch & Fisher, 1998), and the consistently bland flavour of formula may make the infant less willing to try new foods. Formula feeding may thereby reinforce innate preferences for salty and sugary foods.
- Artificially fed infants may have less control over food intake because formula lacks components of human milk (see below) which inhibit appetite and produce satiety.

There is growing evidence that diet in infancy has short- and long-term effects on how the body metabolises food, as well as influencing food intake levels and composition.

- Research in the 1990s showed that the normal energy intake of infants has been considerably overestimated (Dewey et al., 1995). This has resulted in regulatory nutrition standards for infant formulas that will cause overfeeding. Excessive intake of energy and protein in infancy is now a recognised factor in causing rapid early weight gain and altered nutritional programming (Lucas, 1991, 1998, 2000) that increases the risk of obesity in adolescence and adulthood (Baird et al., 2005). Rapid weight gain in early infancy is now also thought to play a key role in adversely programming later health outcomes such as heart disease and diabetes.
- Components in breastmilk (including a complex and dynamic mix of nutrients, hormones, growth factors and fats) play a key role in developing body systems to appropriately regulate food intake, process fats and sugars, and influence fat formation and body weight (Hamosh, 2001). For example, formula fed infants have significantly higher energy intakes than breastfed infants, and feeding triggers different hormonal responses to feeding because formula lacks the various bioactive components in human milk (Lucas et al., 1980). Human milk contains leptin, which controls appetite and satiety as well as energy expenditure, and may perform a counter-regulatory role to insulin in the body (Lyle et al. 2001; Singhal et al., 2002). The dietary fat composition of formula also differs from breastmilk and promotes excessive and abnormal fat cell development (Ailhood & Guesnet, 2004; Koletzko et al., 2001). Commercial infant formula also has a cholesterol and saturated fatty acid content more markedly different from mature breastmilk than the unmodified cows milk used for artificial feeding until the late 1960s (Martin, Ebrahim et al., 2005).

These altered hormone levels and fat concentrations in infancy affect the functioning, growth and development of body organs and tissues, increasing the propensity for fat and glucose metabolism disorders. Studies have found breastfeeding in infancy is associated with reduced chronic disease symptoms (such as high cholesterol levels, blood pressure, insulin resistance, and atherosclerosis) in later life (Ravelli et al., 2000). For example, breastfeeding in full-term infants is associated with lower blood pressure in adolescence and adulthood (Lawlor 2005; Martin, Gunnell & Smith, 2005), while breastfed infants are found to have lower levels of cholesterol and low density lipoproteins, suggesting long-term effects on fatty acid metabolism (Owen et al., 2005). Those breastfed as infants therefore have fewer risk factors for cardiovascular disease and diabetes in later life. Breastfeeding in infancy is likely to reduce the risk of obesity through similar processes to those by which it protects against these other conditions in the metabolic syndrome (Plagemann & Harder, 2005).

Likewise, complex effects of lactation on the maternal body metabolism and endocrine system may explain the 0.6–2.0 kilogram higher postpartum weight retention among formula feeding mothers (Dewey et al., 1993; Ohlin & Rossner, 1990).

'Mass mammary malfunction' from the 1930s

Until World War II, virtually all mothers initiated breastfeeding. High breastfeeding initiation rates were typical in Australian cities early in the 20th century when the usual weaning age was around 9 months. Those now reaching middle age in Australia – those born since the 1950s – are the first generation in history that have not been substantially breastfed in infancy, and those born since around 1970 were the first generation in which use of commercial artificial infant feeding products was widespread.

As historian Janet McCalman (1984) observed in her study of life in Richmond, Victoria, 'the 1930s marked "the beginning of the end of easy breastfeeding" in Australia'. A sharp fall in breastfeeding initiation and increased supplementation occurred around 1942, with recovery after the war. There was then a drastic decline in breastfeeding initiation and duration, which accelerated from the mid-1950s. Breastfeeding rates rose again from the late 1960s, but this was not sustained through the 1980s. There has been no increase in breastfeeding duration since 1985.

FIGURE 1 Long-term trends in breastfeeding in Australia, initiation and full breastfeeding at 3, 6 and 9 months[1]

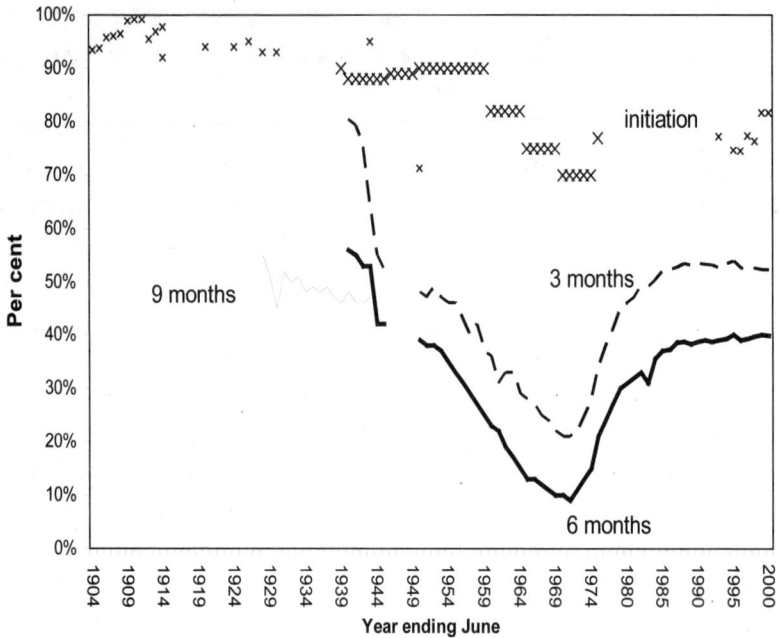

Recent surveys suggest a possible decline in rates of exclusive breastfeeding at 6 months from the 1990s (Gabriel et al., 2005; Hector et al., 2005). Overall, this means that total human milk consumption in Australia has not risen in recent decades.

Just as the earlier fall in breastfeeding had been led by middle-class, educated women (Lund-Adams & Heywood, 1995), so the rise in breastfeeding from the 1970s mainly occurred among those of higher socioeconomic status. Babies from more deprived families typically breastfeed for only a short time, if at all, and are weaned onto formula and solids in the first six months. In 2001, around one in five children from the most disadvantaged families had never been breastfed, twice the likelihood in the most advantaged families

(Australian Institute of Health and Welfare, 2003). This could partly explain why lower socioeconomic groups experience a particularly high prevalence of obesity and its related risk factors.

'Scientific' mothering and 'expert' infant feeding

MEDICAL AUTHORITY AND THE INFANT FOOD MARKET

In the decades after 1900, medical opinion came to play an increasing role in determining infant feeding practices. Mothers themselves increasingly deferred to the opinions of medical and child health 'experts'. This coincided with a growing cultural and medical emphasis on quantifying and measuring the human body as an indicator of both health and morality, which had religious overtones in its search for 'God's rules on earth' (Jutel, 2001). As in the United States, the paediatric profession was also developing strong collaboration with the infant food industry in order to better control infant food quality and marketing practices and to establish the discipline as expert in the 'science' of infant care (Greer & Apple, 1991). Meanwhile difficulties finding suitable wet nurses in Australia, and 'expert' scepticism that modern women could breastfeed successfully (Featherstone, 2001), were reflected in a new public discussion and medical diagnosis of 'lactation failure' (Wolf, 2000).

Medical interest in infant feeding arose from health concerns about new infant feeding products. Although breastfeeding was near-universal, pap or panada (semi-liquid or soft food for infants, such as bread boiled to a pulp and flavoured) was commonly introduced early (Wickes, 1953). New technologies were opening up new market opportunities. From the 1850s, the use of patent infant foods became more widespread as tinned condensed milk and powdered milk became available. Improved transportation and refrigeration had also expanded dairy milk supply in the cities by the 1890s, with dire consequences for the unsafe feeding of infants and children.

By the turn of the century, the growing market in commercial infant foods prompted the Australian medical profession to debate the question of artificial feeding. This led ultimately to medical endorsement of certain products and brands as 'safe' for infants from 6 months. Influential research in the United States in the late 1920s found that newborns fed evaporated milk gained more weight than other infants, contributing to medical acceptance of artificial feeding. The success of the safe milk campaigns convinced paediatricians there that breastfeeding was largely irrelevant to infant health. By the 1930s, commercial formula feeding was generally accepted by the medical professional as 'safe' (Greer & Apple, 1991).

'SCIENTIFIC' MOTHERING AND HEALTHY WEIGHT GAIN

The focus on measurement and science also permeated the infant welfare movement emerging in the early decades of the 20th century, and this movement was increasingly influential from the 1920s. It also placed mothers under the supervision of health professional 'experts', devaluing and undermining women's own expertise and confidence on infant care and feeding (Reiger, 1991). Beliefs and practices promoted the desirability of fat babies, despite the greater health risks that this could promote.

Strongly influenced by 'Truby King' ideologies and practices, the movement placed near-religious emphasis on 'feeding and sleeping by the clock' – a baby reared on Truby King's rules would obey the Ten Commandments (Mein Smith, 1988, 1997).[2] According to King, 'the main cause of modern bodily unfitness and inefficiency lies with our women, and is not due to indifference on their part but to lack of the necessary knowledge ... [of] the laws of healthy living'.

From the 1930s, the 'scientific' infant care practices advocated through the clinics also promoted the belief that a heavy infant is a healthy infant. Weight gain became the main focus of infant health. Test weighing scales, available more widely from the 1920s, were the symbol of 'scientific' infant care. Perceived 'insufficient' weight gain led many mothers to introduce artificial baby milks on the advice of health professionals, or to abandon breastfeeding due to 'inadequate milk' (Thorley, 2003).

Throughout the postwar era there was also widespread use of infant age-weight charts, developed in the United States during the 1950s. These were based on formula fed populations, which, as noted earlier, have now been found to overestimate normal weight gain of infants – a WHO study of 8000 exclusively breastfed infants found that normal weight gain is both highly variable within populations and on average around 7 per cent less than suggested by current growth charts (WHO, 2006). Combined with the centrality of weight gain in infant growth monitoring and feeding since the 1920s, this suggests many adequately nourished infants were weaned unnecessarily from breastfeeding due to anxieties provoked by inaccurate charts and excessive infant weight gain standards.

THE ROLE OF SURPLUS DAIRY PRODUCTION

Australia's postwar market for commercial infant foods was expanded by cheaper supplies and new approaches to marketing and distribution, as it has more recently in developing countries (Post and Smith, 1988). Marketing and promotion of commercial infant formula translated new production opportunities created by improved transport technologies and dairying productivity into a mass market for commercial infant food from the 1950s.

Several supply-related factors stimulated more vigorous promotion and marketing of dairy products generally in Australia after World War II. A dramatic increase in world dairy production occurred in the post-war decades due to improved farm practices, new technology and European agricultural policies. Government land development and irrigation policies expanded the Australian dairy industry. By the mid-1960s, the output of milk per dairy cow in Australia was around 476 gallons (1800 litres) per cow, compared to below 300 gallons (1100 litres) per cow around the turn of the century (Australian Bureau of Statistics, 1969, p. 907). Powdered milk production for the three years ended 1958–59 was more than five times higher than before the war. Growth in butter and cheese production also left large domestic skim milk and whey surpluses needing a market. Manufacture of infant formula became a convenient and growing outlet for these surpluses. As birth rates in Western Europe and North America declined from the 1950s and market saturation loomed, infant formula manufacturers sought new export markets (Ebrahim, 1978).

With recovery from the after-effects of the war and the end of import controls, competition in the Australian infant food market intensified from the mid-1950s.

THE EFFECTS OF COMPETITION FOR MARKET SHARE

Most mothers who were artificially feeding in Australia at that time had used either home-modified fresh or powdered cows milk, evaporated milk or Nestlé's Lactogen (Thorley, 2003). Until the 1950s, there had been little competition in the small Australian market for commercial infant milk formulas. Nestlé held the dominant position, although New Zealand's Glaxo and Karicare products were also available. Direct advertising to mothers was not common. However, from around the mid-1950s there were two new entrants to the Australian infant formula market. United States pharmaceutical companies Mead Johnson, Wyeth and Abbott Ross marketed their products in active competition with Nestlé, bringing to the task their long experience in marketing pharmaceutical products to health professionals and institutions.

TABLE 1 Trends in per capita consumption of milk products used for infant feeding, Australia 1939–99

Year ended June	Infants and invalids food, kg per capita	Condensed, concentrated, evaporated milk, kg per capita	Powdered milk, kg per capita
1939	0.5	2.0	1.2
1949	0.6	3.4	1.5
1959	1.0	4.1	1.1
1971	1.0	6.8	4.8
1979	1.2	2.9	2.2
1989	1.4	1.8	1.9
1999	na	0.8	1.5

The scramble for market share drastically increased the size of the market for commercial formula by reducing the 'market' for breastmilk. Together, table 1 and figure 2 show Australian per capita consumption of all processed milk products used for infant feeding[3] since 1939. They show:

- a substantial acceleration in the sale and consumption of specialised infant milk products beginning in the 1950s;
- peak per capita consumption of condensed, evaporated and powdered milk products (commonly – although not exclusively – used in artificial infant feeding) in the early 1970s, when breastfeeding rates were at their nadir; and
- a continued rise in sales of infant milk products throughout the 1980s and 1990s.

FIGURE 2 Annual sales of infant formula

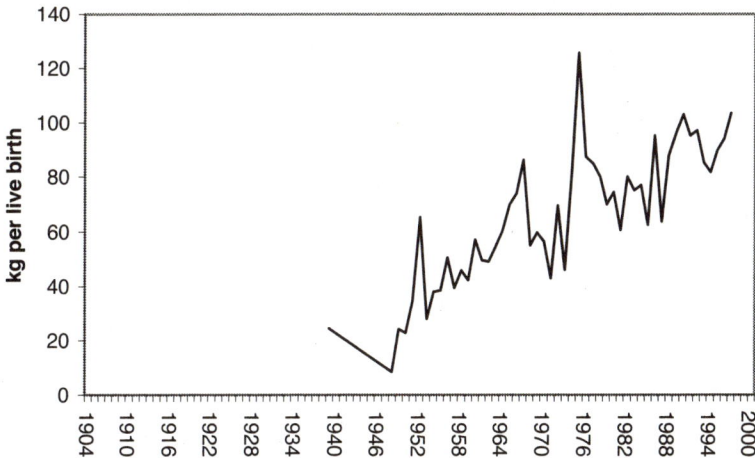

'SCIENTIFIC' MATERNITY CARE SERVICES

Ironically, the major new distribution and marketing outlet for these new commercial infant feeding products was the health system. Hospital-based and medicated childbirth increased in Australia from the 1930s and was nearly universal by 1945, and by World War II, infant welfare clinic attendance was widespread even in remote areas (Reiger, 1985). There was pressure from doctors and nurses to breastfeed. However, practices imposed by this widespread system of supposedly 'scientific' institutionalised care interfered with the establishment of lactation and successful maintenance of breastfeeding in several generations of mothers and babies (Mein Smith, 1997; Reiger, 2001; Thorley, 2003), and resulted in almost universal artificial feeding of Australian infants by the mid- to late-1960s.

In the years following World War II, most mothers received analgesia during childbirth, and it was common for mother and baby to be separated for many hours after birth. Widespread use of analgesia during labour and delivery, and separation of mother and infant are now recognised to harm establishment of breastfeeding and maternal bonding (Enkin et al., 1995; WHO Division of Child Health and Development, 1998). From the 1940s, 'after giving birth in large hospitals women had little to do with their babies, who were whisked off to nurseries and they to wards' (Reiger, 2001, p. 32). Although a few doctors and midwives maintained the early custom of putting the baby to the breast soon after delivery, this was no longer normal practice after the war. Many mothers and babies were in any case affected by medication. Mothers usually waited for several hours, and sometimes even two to three days, for their babies to be brought to them from the central nursery for the first feed. Mothers of premature infants waited even longer. The result was that many babies were given either glucose and water, or formula, before even starting breastfeeding.

In the early postnatal period infants were universally cared for in hospital nurseries where regimented and highly restrictive feeding regimes were imposed. These practices in infant care are now recognised to hinder responsiveness to infant feeding cues and the establishment of good milk supply. Restricting the number and/or duration of feeds risks excessive postpartum weight loss in the baby, and contributes to breast engorgement and related problems for the mother, often resulting in early cessation of breastfeeding. The use of dummies, bottles, teats and test weighing (weighing of babe before and after feeds) also makes it more likely that breastfeeding will be abandoned in the early postnatal period.

From the 1940s, newborns were kept in central nurseries with strictly scheduled feeding times – only two minutes of feeding were allowed on each breast every six hours in the early days postpartum, and up to ten minutes a side until discharge from hospital (Thorley, 2002). Mothers were then admonished to adhere to feeding every four hours and give no feeds within an eight-hour period overnight. Even mothers with engorgement were not allowed to put babies to the breast outside of scheduled feeding times. Test weighing was the usual procedure, and mothers of babies deemed underweight were instructed to give top-up feeds of home-modified animal milks or infant formulas. Dummies were also widely used in the nurseries. According to an obstetrician of the time, 'babies in nurseries, four hourly feeding, test weighed and complementary feeds, particularly at night, [were] *absolute* routine, in *all* hospitals' (Reiger, 2001, p. 59). Some health authorities also insisted on mothers giving babies bottled fruit juice from around a month after birth, and supplementation with bottled water was commonly recommended to provide supposedly necessary additional fluids or to stretch the time between feeds.

Lack of skilled, sensitive support for breastfeeding by health professionals and the mother's family and community also harms breastfeeding. Mothers during the 1940s and 1950s were told to scrub their nipples with a nailbrush to toughen them up and were commonly recommended creams or other treatments for sore nipples that have since been shown to be harmful, or at best ineffective, in preventing cross-infection or pain on breastfeeding.

Far from reflecting 'scientific' knowledge, much of the infant feeding advice authoritatively provided to new mothers was based on the authority of gurus of the Australian infant welfare movement such as Truby King. According to Thorley (2002, p. 26):

> 'Scientific mothering' was a misnomer for the practices of the time, for it would appear that measurement and time-keeping masqueraded as 'science', while the authority of what had been practised for several decades made the system immune to incursions from studies or contrary opinions published in medical journals accessible to Australia.

Given these institutional practices and 'expert' opinion, it is a testimony to Australian mothers' fortitude and commitment to breastfeeding that even in the mid-1960s, more than two-thirds commenced breastfeeding and one in five fully breastfed when their baby was 3 months (see figure 1).

MASS MARKETING THROUGH THE HEALTH SYSTEM

A marketing strategy aimed mainly at physicians had characterised formula marketing in the United States from the 1930s. This was after the medical profession and the industry had formalised their collaboration in the development and advertising of artificial infant foods (Greer & Apple, 1991).

A similarly 'beneficial, reciprocal relationship' had also been established with Australian hospitals during the 1940s by Nestlé and later the Carnation Company. As a consequence, manufacturers were well placed to take advantage of new mothers' uncertainties and their struggles with milk supply that arose from the restrictive breastfeeding practices of the era.

By the 1950s, distribution of company promotional materials by maternity staff gave marketing access to virtually all Australian mothers. Infant formula manufacturers had long produced free booklets on parenting and infant feeding; these were widely distributed through the hospitals. These were slanted towards product promotion and reinforced adherence to the rigid regimes that worked against breastfeeding. For example, Nestlé's booklet warned mothers of newborns that they should immediately obtain a set of test-feeding scales to measure breastmilk intake, as 'it is very necessary to find out whether baby is getting sufficient food and this is the only way of doing it with any degree of accuracy' (Thorley, 2003, p. 70).

The direct advertising of commercial formulas to health professionals increased rapidly from the 1950s as Nestlé sought to protect its market dominance from incursions by Mead Johnson and other suppliers. For example, by 1965, the number of advertisements for infant feeding related products and advertising of infant formula and milks in the *Medical Journal of Australia* was almost five times higher than for 1950–55. The growth of direct advertising to doctors is indicated by figure 3.

In the more competitive market environment of the late-1950s, hospitals and health professionals were also enlisted directly in aggressive marketing practices, such as free distribution of formulas to hospitals and to mothers at discharge, as well as direct advertising (Thorley, 2003). By the mid-1970s, it is said, hospitals had become 'display cases' for the promotion of artificial feeding

FIGURE 3 Advertising of commercial baby milks and formulas in the *Medical Journal of Australia*, 1950–85

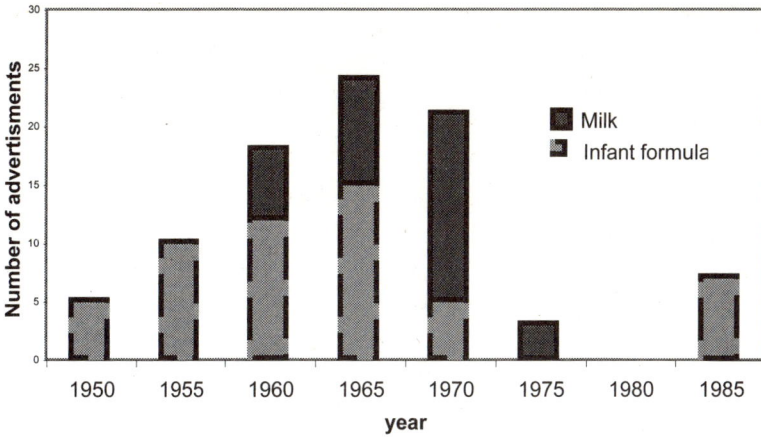

(Lund-Adams & Heywood 1995). Over this same period, direct advertising to mothers also increased dramatically. For example, the number of advertisements for infant foods and milks in the *Australian Women's Weekly* multiplied seven-fold in the decade from 1955 (see figure 4), with the number of these magazine advertisements peaking in the early 1970s. Marketing messages had by then shifted from the mother who 'couldn't' breastfeed to the one who 'chose' not to, and emphasis had moved from building mothers' trust that the product was safe, and developed by scientific experts, to assertions that the product was as good as or better than mothers milk. Reduced breastfeeding duration is a predictable result of unsupportive health institution policies including, for example, the commercial discharge packs or free samples (Enkin et al., 1995; WHO Division of Child Health and Development, 1998) that were a feature of this era.

Figure 1 shows breastfeeding at 3 months falling from around 50 per cent to 20 per cent between 1949 and 1970, and table 1 shows continually rising sales trends for commercial infant milk products commencing in the mid-1950s.

The continuing rise in consumption of commercial formula from the early 1970s despite rising breastfeeding initiation is worthy of further comment. It largely reflects the replacement

FIGURE 4 Advertising of commercial baby milks and formulas in the *Australian Women's Weekly*, Australia, 1950–85

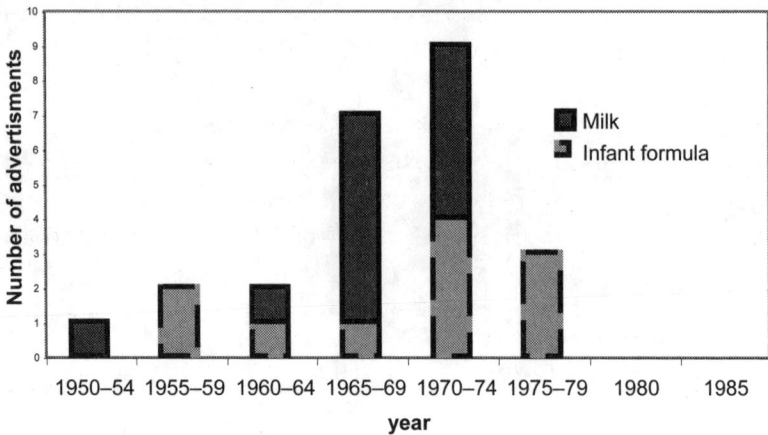

of home-prepared formulas by commercial formulas since the 1970s. More recently it is likely to reflect expanded marketing and sales of formulas targeting mothers of older infants ('follow-on' or 'toddler' formulas). These emerged in the mid-1980s as a strategic response to the WHO Code, which constrains marketing of products for younger infants (Greer & Apple, 1991; Minchin, 1998). Promotion of these products is increasingly used to 'cross-market' other branded infant food products. The marketing of these formula products has become increasingly aggressive in the Australian market in recent years, as competition intensifies. Most recently, this reflects the provision of a Commonwealth government subsidy for market entry of a new 'organic' formula (Truss, 2004).

Combined with evidence in figures 3 and 4 on advertising activity, the above suggests that between the mid-1950s and 1970 companies promoting use of formula products were competing not just for 'market share' in a market of fixed size, but to grow the market for commercial infant milk products. That is, they were promoting commercial products in a market where they were competing against mothers milk and breastfeeding. A similar conclusion may be drawn regarding the effects on breastfeeding of recent competition to promote new 'follow-on' and 'toddler' formulas.

The return to breastfeeding from the early 1970s reflected mothers themselves reclaiming expertise on breastfeeding, with the growing influence and activism of community-based groups such as the Nursing Mothers' Association (Reiger, 2001; Smibert, 1988). Likewise, in New Zealand and Norway the return to breastfeeding reflected the growing strength of community-based breastfeeding support and activism (Austveg & Sundby, 1995; Ryan & Beresford, 1997).

Not until the mid-1980s did Australian governments take steps to constrain industry and health services' advertising and promotion of artificial infant feeding. Responding to the 1981 WHO International Code on the Marketing of Breastmilk Substitutes (WHO, 1981), the Commonwealth government facilitated a voluntary industry agreement (Marketing Agreement on Infant Formula [MAIF]) among manufacturers and importers of infant formula in 1985. To further the objectives of the WHO Code, the National Health and Medical Research Council (NHMRC) also developed and published infant feeding guidelines for health workers (NHMRC, 2003).

The MAIF excludes retailers, and a wide range of products covered by the WHO Code such as infant cereals, juices, yogurts, and feeding implements, bottles, dummies and teats. Industry has also interpreted the agreement to exclude so-called 'follow-on' and 'toddler' formulas. Several significant manufacturers have not signed the agreement, which in any case is unenforceable. Likewise, NHMRC guidelines for health workers, which encompass matters such as conflict of interest and receipt of commercial sponsorship and gifts, rely on voluntary compliance.

FEMALE LABOUR MARKET TRENDS: COMPETITION FOR MOTHERS' TIME

As inflexible working arrangements and attitudes present barriers to breastfeeding mothers, greater employment opportunities and rising remuneration for market work potentially 'competes' with breastfeeding through the competition for mothers' time. As breastfeeding requires a considerable time commitment from the mother, at least in the early months, rising workforce participation among new mothers might represent a growing market opportunity for commercial infant milk formula. Was the decline in breastfeeding from the mid-1950s due to economic factors such

FIGURE 5 Female labour force participation rates, 1954–2003

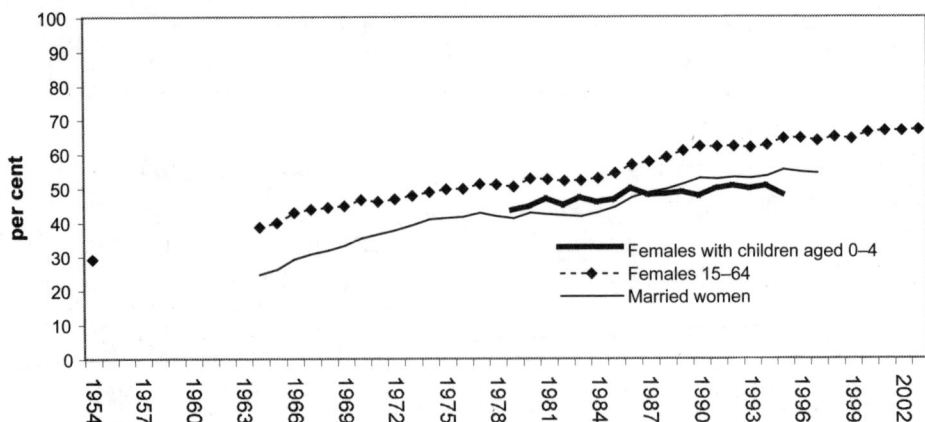

as women's rising participation in the labour market, rather than commercial marketing and health institutional practices?

Figure 5 shows labour force participation rates for women since the mid-1950s. During this period, married women withdrew from the workforce, and social and institutional barriers, including lack of childcare services, taxation incentives for dependent wives, and policies of compulsory resignation on marriage, discouraged women's employment. Until the mid-1960s labour force participation rates were typically around 30 per cent for women 25–40 years of age. Rising participation in the early 1960s accelerated from 1971. By the mid-1990s, around two-thirds of women of childbearing age were in employment. The remarkable growth in female labour force participation since the 1950s was mainly higher part-time participation by married women. Nevertheless, until 1976, women of peak childbearing age (20–40 years) were generally less likely to be in the workforce. This being the case, rising labour market participation by mothers of infants during the 1950s and early 1960s, even if rising, is unlikely to have been common enough to account for the 20–30 percentage point decline in breastfeeding initiation and prevalence during the decade from 1955 (see figure 1).

Likewise, it was in the early 1970s – not during the 1950s and 1960s – that the relative profitability of paid work for mothers

FIGURE 6 Female—male earnings ratio, 1954—2003

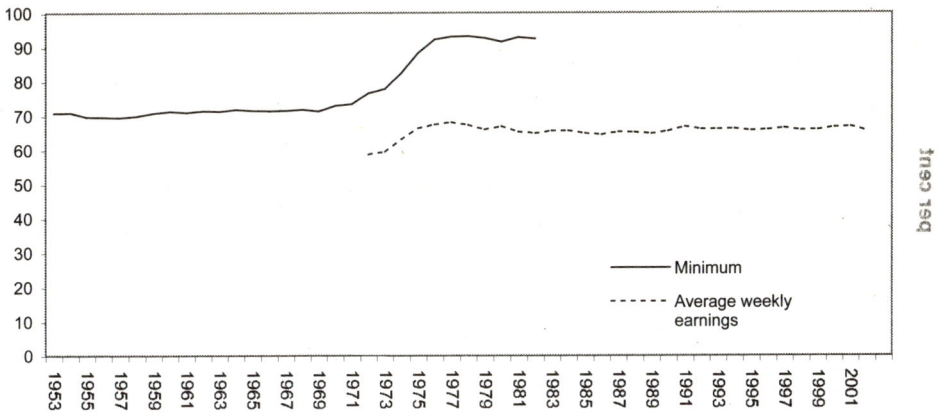

FIGURE 6 Female—male earnings ratio, 1954—2003

increased most markedly (see figure 6). This reflected tightening labour market conditions in the late 1960s and the equal pay decisions of the Commonwealth Conciliation and Arbitration Commission in the early 1970s. Trends to equal pay for women after World War II may have increased the 'opportunity cost' of breastfeeding. However, this occurred when breastfeeding rates were increasing, rather than during the 1960s when breastfeeding declined the most, suggesting that labour market incentives were not the main factor reducing breastfeeding during the 1960s.

There has been little substantial improvement in breastfeeding since the mid-1980s, despite slight improvement in initiation (see figure 1). This coincides with both the rise in female labour force rewards and participation (see figures 5 and 6) and the continued rise in per capita sales and consumption of commercial infant milk products. The latter is likely to be partly due to growing use of 'follow-on' and 'toddler' formulas – which are marketed to mothers of infants over 6 months of age (see figure 2) – as well as to declining exclusive breastfeeding before 6 months.

The above suggests that labour market competition for mothers' time does not explain the rapid growth in artificial infant feeding between 1955 and 1972, even if it may help explain the lack of improvement in breastfeeding duration since the mid-1980s.

Conclusion: Did marketing matter?

Those who view obesity as simply a matter of eating too much and exercising too little might well consider the case of infant feeding, and the marketing of infant foods. Is it reasonable to argue that breastfeeding is simply a matter of individual choice, and that individuals determine their own weight destiny, when the institutional and market environment can be shown to produce such dramatic changes in infant feeding practices?

Artificial infant feeding is a risk factor for obesity, yet for several decades, Australia's health care system and industry regulatory framework provided an environment that has not only permitted but facilitated commercial promotion of unhealthy – in hindsight, experimental – infant feeding practices. Although there remain significant uncertainties about exactly how infant feeding affects the metabolism during infancy and in later life, findings that nutrition in early life may have major biological effects on later health and development present a major challenge to current infant nutrition policies, standards and practices, and emphasise the need to refocus on long-term health and development, rather than infant weight gain (Singhal et al., 2004). Past policies and feeding recommendations focused on achieving weight gain have not been scientifically based. Indeed, according to one of the world's leading experimental researchers in infant nutrition:

> For normal infants, let alone fetuses, there is hardly a nutritional management policy or recommended dietary allowance that could be adequately scientifically defended in terms of its beneficial effects later in life. (Lucas, 1998)

This conclusion reinforces the observation from two decades ago that 'artificial feeding of infants is, in fact, the largest uncontrolled *in vivo* experiment in human history' (Minchin, 1985). Few parents are aware of this when making critical decisions about infant feeding.

Notably, the public health sector itself has been, and still is, complicit in the decline in breastfeeding; disruptive health care regimes and unsound 'expert' recommendations undermined mothers' autonomy, confidence and skills and led to reduced breastfeeding, increased formula feeding, and overfeeding of artificially fed infants. Although 'fat' babies were, and continue to be, encouraged, 'fat' children and adults are now seen as a significant public health problem.

Although more mothers now initiate breastfeeding than they did in the 1960s, the consumption of artificial infant formula continues to increase. The latest figures suggest exclusive breastfeeding at 6 months is declining. As shown above, this is in part because governments and the health system continue to facilitate promotion and marketing of commercial infant feeding products. Continuing health system and regulatory failure to implement WHO and NHMRC infant feeding recommendations perpetuate problems of dated and inaccurate health professional advice and misleading infant food labelling and thereby contribute to excessive weight gain, early introduction of solids and reduced breastfeeding. In the absence of effective enforcement of codes of practice for health professionals and industry, infant formula companies also continue to promote obesogenic infant feeding practices to health professionals in the guise of 'education'.

Hospitals and health professionals continue to engage in inappropriate conflict of interest activities in receiving free supplies, sponsorship, gifts or inducements, contrary to the WHO Code of Marketing of Breastmilk Substitutes and which ought to be contrary to professional ethical standards and codes of conduct. This occurs despite growing public unease at pervasive medical and research alliances with the pharmaceutical industry (Moynihan & Henry, 2006). Those who see no harm in these practices could well reflect on whether they would have the same view if it were tobacco companies providing gifts and funding to health professionals engaged in lung cancer work.

As well as showing how commercial and professional vested interests took over as 'experts' on infant feeding in the past several decades, this story of baby food marketing and fat highlights how an increasingly competitive market in commercial infant feeding products led to aggressive product promotion, and less breastfeeding. Marketing also shifted artificial infant feeding from unsatisfactory home-made mixtures based on unmodified cows milk, to more complex but possibly more obesogenic commercial formulas since the 1970s. As has been shown for tobacco, competition to protect or gain market share expands the size of the market and does not just shift consumers between brands (Chaloupka et al., 2005).

This story also points to the possibility that the epidemic of artificial feeding from the 1950s and the growing use of formula in artificial feeding since the 1970s could help explain the current epidemic of obesity, notably among infants and children from low SES background whose exposure to artificial feeding is still high, and the expanding cohort of 40+ year old adults whose food metabolism has been shaped by the widespread premature weaning of infants from breastmilk.

This chapter has also considered economic factors that might explain increased consumer demand for commercial infant foods, including changes in relative costs (such as trends in mothers' potential labour market earnings). Such trends could make breastfeeding more or less costly to women in terms of lost earnings. However, it is shown here that changing workforce opportunities for mothers do not explain the vast expansion in the commercial infant food market from 1955.

To the contrary, evidence from the successful promotion of artificial infant feeding through the health system during the 1950s and 1960s shows that food promotion and marketing is what matters. That is to say, marketing and promotion is important to eating behaviour, and mothers milk competes in the 'market' on highly unfavourable terms against commercial infant food products. This emphasises the need for governments and health professional organisations to introduce effective restraints on the promotion and marketing of artificial feeding for infants and young children, including of 'follow-on' and 'toddler' formulas, and other commercial substitutes for breastmilk, including infant foods and drinks.

---

1   Victorian infant health clinic data on rates of 'full' breastfeeding at 3, 6 and (for the 1920s) 9 months provide the main information for the period from 1927 to the present (Mortenson, 2001). Data from mothers attending clinics suffer from self-selection bias and may not show the true prevalence of breastfeeding. Nevertheless, this series, combined

with earlier data from Sydney (Armstrong, 1939), Brisbane (Siskind et al., 1993) and central Melbourne (Mein Smith, 1997), can be argued to provide a reasonable indication of broad trends and periods of major change during the century.

2 Truby King was a very influential New Zealand infant welfare authority who claimed his infant care prescriptions were responsible for that country's low infant mortality rate, a claim that has been challenged by recent historical analysis (Mein Smith, 1997).

3 This classification also includes invalids food, although it is mainly infant milk formula. 'Invalids' included mothers who were encouraged by health professionals and the infant food companies to drink milk-based dietary supplements, including artificial baby milks supposedly to increase their milk supply. See Thorley (2002).

SIN#7:
THE ENVIRONMENT OF
COMPETING AUTHORITIES

Saturated with choice

Jane Dixon and Christine Winter

Until recently, able-bodied people in receipt of modest incomes did not give diet or physical activity a second thought. Food security was the norm, and physical activity was built into daily life as well as being pursued through informal sports or games outside the eight-hour working day or the school day. As obligatory physical exercise diminishes due to automation, much physical activity must now be intentionally undertaken. People rely on more organised forms of exercise such as gym use, walking groups or club sports rather than incidental and spontaneous activity. Such exercise requires motivation, planning and (sometimes) money, so individuals without these attributes are excluded. In the past physical activity produced goods or services as part of paid work, personal transport or domestic activities, but exercise is now typically economically unproductive (for example, running), and is sometimes costly (for example, the gym).

A similar case can be made in relation to diet. Food is no longer about satiety, ritual and pleasure but is more culturally loaded than in the past: it now represents a pathway to individual status and identity and a reflection of moral worth (the sociology of vegetarianism offers ample testimony of this point).

Building on earlier chapters, we focus on the recent genesis of changed cultural dispositions towards the two behaviours that underpin weight gain: physical activity and food consumption. Denniss (this volume) describes modern citizens as hyper-consumers, people engrossed in their consumption activities. This chapter proposes that many modern consumers are cultural omnivores: compared with their parents they have a relatively wide range of tastes, which are often transitory in keeping with the fashions encouraged by commodity and knowledge producers. An appreciation for relentless market-based consumption is not an inherited or innate state of being (see chapters by Denniss and Smith, this volume). Professional marketers expend considerable effort to foster the desire for novelty and to experiment with the latest commercial offerings. Indeed, Australians are frequently described as 'early adopters', embracing novel technologies such as the home computer and mobile phone before other nations.

The question this chapter addresses is: Where does this impulse for omnivorous consumption come from? Does it reflect a young, multicultural nation at ease with diverse traditions? Or is it an economically rational response to the smorgasbord of marketplace offerings? Both explanations are plausible.

The rise of the omnivorous and anxious consumer

A further explanation receives attention from the fields of food sociology and physical activity research. There is growing speculation that flexible, transient and omnivorous approaches to diet and exercise are accompanied by a pervasive sense of anxiety about what advice to follow and which advice-givers to trust. It has been suggested that the more anxious and confused people are, the more susceptible they are to experimenting with the latest, unproven approach to exercise, diets and weight loss (Katz, 2005).

Some years ago, French sociologist Claude Fischler (1988) described how the human biological need for a range of food types inevitably arouses anxiety. He referred to this condition as 'omnivore's paradox'; and he noted that anxiety was flourishing in modern societies due to the enormous diversity of available food choices. He also described how the global movement of foodstuffs and cuisines fuelled consumer ignorance about food, including its origins, its uses and its social and cultural significance. This culinary alienation led eaters to consult an ever-wider range of sources of advice in the search for security, resulting in what he termed the 'nutritional cacophony' of competing experts. Fischler's arguments continue to resonate with developments in Australia's food system, and they equally apply to the physical activity cacophony.

This chapter concentrates on the environment of multiple sources of conflicting advice about what to eat, how much to exercise, and more generally how 'to be' a modern citizen. We contend that omnivorous and anxious Australians are subject to a proliferating range of products as well as numerous authorities competing to guide decisions about healthy diets and exercise. As a result, increasing numbers of people are either overtly repudiating expert advice and experimenting with their own approaches and solutions (some effective and others ineffective), or are so thoroughly confused as to be paralysed into inaction.

In the next section we consider in more depth the origins of consumer anxiety, attributing it to four factors: a crisis of legitimacy regarding authority figures; the market's promotion of charismatic authority; the market's promotion of individual choice (a virtue requiring expert guidance); and the emergence of industry self-regulation, with the subsequent commercialisation of advice. Examples are provided of how these factors influence patterns of physical activity and diet. We conclude by discussing how omnivorous consumption by confused citizens can produce weight gain.

Origins of the anxious consumer

For four decades, social theorists have been writing about 'the crisis of legitimacy' afflicting modern, democratic governments and other institutions. As a result of political scandals, financial debt and unjust policies, governments are no longer automatically accepted as the major, independent guardian of the public good. Other symbols of strength and guidance have also suffered their own legitimation crises: the Church, the monarchy, the corporation and the elite private school. Diminished legitimacy is accompanied by a loss in the persuasive powers of the ideas promoted by those institutions, and by the active resistance and subversion of their ideas by a cynical public or an 'unmanageable consumer' (Gabriel & Lang, 1995).

Among the more recent casualties to have lost their aura of authority are the professionals including teachers, doctors, lawyers and social workers. The unquestioned legitimacy of scientists has also come to an end, in part due to well-publicised frauds and in part because of the media's appetite to assume the role of knowledge broker. No longer content as the gatherer and disseminator of news, the media promote high profile individuals and organisations, often with little content knowledge, to interpret world events and the latest discoveries (Pileggi & Patton, 2003, p. 318). The findings of single studies that either have a shock factor or offer unbridled hope in terms of a cure are commonly reported without critical interpretation. However, the conclusions from individual pieces of research are invariably short-lived and the subject of refutation by other studies, leaving the population wondering whom they can trust. This was well illustrated by an article in *Science* magazine devoted to questions about the quality of the science emanating from the Centers for Disease Control (CDC), the United States government body charged with tracking the nation's health. In the space of a few months in 2004, CDC staff had published three articles variously estimating annual death toll due to obesity to be 400 000, 365 000 and 112 000. Dissent among CDC scientists regarding the best way to calculate the figures became a very public feud. The lack of agreement, and successive lowering of the estimates, was seized upon by the food industry which announced opportunistically that obesity was probably not a significant risk factor for death or disease (Couzin, 2005, p. 770).

Not only are authorities being scrutinised and commented upon in an unprecedented way, but the nature of authority is being transformed. Dixon (2003) has argued that charismatic authority (which derives from possessing extraordinary qualities) is eclipsing both traditional and bureaucratic/legal authority. Charismatic figures include sports stars, film stars, mass media celebrities such as Oprah Winfrey, and rich and famous entrepreneurs. Journalists and government leaders seek out their opinions and policy prescriptions often before they canvass the opinions of expert academics or policy analysts. In one notable example, the 'celebrity chef' Jamie Oliver advised the British government on how to change children's diets through transforming the operations of school canteens. Jamie's influence over canteen policies has extended to Australia and New Zealand in a way that public health experts have not.

Indeed, it is now commonplace for commercial firms to seek celebrity endorsement of products and services, so that television viewers and lifestyle magazine readers see record-breaking swimmers like Ian Thorpe advertising breakfast cereal and watches, respected actors like Sam Neill promoting red meat, or the archetypal charismatic businessman Richard Branson extolling the merits of a brand of suitcase. The emergence of celebrity endorsement has been made possible by the dominant role of the mass media in the diffusion of knowledge.

However, the new producers of knowledge do not have to be rich, famous or gifted individuals; firms can invent their own figures of authority, as has happened with Ronald McDonald, the creation of the McDonald's hamburger chain. Now no longer content to assist the curative side of health through subsidising Ronald McDonald Houses attached to major children's hospitals, Ronald, who appears in public most often as a cartoon character, has become a preventer of ill-health. Recently, the corporation made him its 'chief happiness officer', and an 'ambassador for an active, balanced lifestyle', who will visit American schools to talk about the importance of physical activity (Simon, 2005). In this undertaking Ronald will, with the backing of the world's most successful fast food chain, dispense advice about health and happiness. In effect, the solemn and bureaucratic authority of the teacher is displaced by the charismatic authority of the corporate clown. By doing his good works for health and happiness in the vicinity of esteemed institutions such as children's hospitals and primary schools, Ronald acquires serious, quasi-scientific intent; which in turn imbues the giant commercial operator with a moral authority in the area of public health.

While the crisis of legitimacy surrounding once-dominant authority figures and the rise of charismatic authorities are relatively recent phenomena, the third factor contributing to consumer confusion and anxiety has been a long time in the making. The mantra of consumer choice as a hallmark of social and economic progress was fostered by the earliest supermarket chains in the 1920s (Humphery, 1998). The size of these stores meant they could stock numerous alternative product lines, much as department stores had done for some decades. In its quest to attract customers away from its major competitor, the small 'mom and pop' store, it was the supermarket that was responsible for demanding product diversity from suppliers.

Promoting choice has had significant implications for both producers and consumers. Producers have had to introduce new product lines with increasing frequency. For consumers, the rigours of exercising choice have encouraged the evolution of consumer-support sectors, including home economics, nutrition education, life science and health promotion. At various times in the last 80 years, each of these mainly scientifically based sources of information has been important to the education of the house wife, shopper, parent and health-conscious person. Commercial firms have also played a part in educating 'Mrs Housewife', 'Junior Consumer', 'Mr Fitness' as the sections that follow show. These firms need not be old, large, household names, although many are. Individuals, operating from home or in a suburban business setting, are selling their services as a 'lifecoach', image consultant or personal trainer: the person paid to teach others how to acquire good habits and make strategic choices among all of life's distractions and opportunities. In an era of autonomous citizens who believe they are creating their own life trajectory, the lifecoach is the successor to the guru, teacher, guide, mentor and psychoanalyst of the previous four decades. Rather than spending days, months and years finding the answer from within, the time-pressured response to self-improvement is to hire an expert, ideally one who embodies the qualities being sought.

This proliferation of advisors is amplified many times by the deregulated oversight of responsibilities for public safety and public health. For example, the large supermarket chains have assumed responsibility to manage hazards arising between their farm suppliers and store shelves. Food processors, the fitness industry and the advertising industry are covered by voluntary codes of conduct as well as minimal oversight from government-based consumer bodies. To signal their regulatory efforts, industry groups develop symbols of quality, codes of practice, industry standards and benchmarks to communicate with customers about the value and integrity of what they produce and sell. Industry self-regulation has introduced a plethora of commercial actors as authority figures, and in the process has commercialised many forms of advice.

Charting transitions in authority, multiplication of advice and the role of the market

Thus far we have argued that there is a discernible transition to multiple, competing authorities, including the advent of charismatic market-based authorities, which contribute to consumer confusion and anxiety. The following sections touch on how this trend, alongside the market's promotion of choice and the commercialisation of advice about how to exercise choice, is reflected in the physical activity and food and nutrition areas. We also illustrate the operation of hybrid forms of authority where market-based actors forge alliances with scientific, government and professional bodies who agree to provide what are called 'third-party endorsements'. This form of indirect marketing is far more persuasive than product advertising sponsored by the firm that stands to gain from the sale of the good or service (Dixon & Banwell, 2004; Nestle, 2002). Thus, it is not surprising that firms like McDonald's are shifting their marketing activities away from direct product advertising to indirect marketing, including sponsoring the highly popular children's program 'Sesame Street', as well as Nickelodeon's 'Playful Parent' series encouraging parent–child play time (Lang et al., 2006).

Physical activity

THE FITNESS INDUSTRY: FROM ANTI-AUTHORITY
TO CHARISMATIC AUTHORITY

One response to the crisis of authority of the late 1960s was an increased longing for 'getting in touch with oneself', a belief that changed people will change the world, and that self-reliance was more effective than expert advice: a *zeitgeist* which seeped from counterculture movements into mainstream society. Critique of, disappointment with, and even disillusionment with traditional authorities spilled over from the political arena into areas of health and fitness (Rader, 1991, p. 257). Specifically, disillusionment with technology and modern medicine during the 1960s and 1970s provided a springboard for the modern fitness trend, and still plays a role in the industry's appeal especially to baby boomers. As Glassner (1989, p. 182) noted, fitness activities provided people with an escape from the disenchantment they were experiencing in relation to 'perceived shortcomings' of modern culture.

The fitness movement, which quickly became the fitness industry, received renewed impetus from the cardiovascular crisis because lifestyle change was widely seen as having more to offer than Western medical intervention (Rader, 1991, pp. 256–58). Just as self-reliance and self-help were transformed from marginal values and lifestyles to mainstream commercial commodities, so was fitness. It seems befitting that Jane Fonda, anti-Vietnam symbol, became one of the earliest icons of the commercialised alternative lifestyle movement, through selling 'aerobics'. The Jane Fonda aerobics videos also had a major impact on Australian fitness habits: in 2002, aerobics was second only to 'walking for exercise' as the most popular general participation sport for women in Australia and the fourth most popular for men (Australian Bureau of Statistics [ABS], 2006b, p. 22).

Viewing the Fonda videos illuminates how altered views of authority accompanied the change of 'fitness' from counterculture to industry. In trying to understand the paradoxical entanglement of self-empowerment with a longing for guidance, Kegan and

Morse (1988) argued that aerobics initially promised self-empowerment but many popular versions of aerobics, where the viewer was asked to copy the movements of a leader (like Fonda), did not fulfil this promise. Instead of negating or challenging outside authority, they reaffirmed it. Analysing Fonda's lack of physical skills, Kegan and Morse argued that Fonda's authority stemmed not from her expertise in exercise but her celebrity status.

MARKET PROMOTION OF INDIVIDUAL CHOICE AND EXPERT GUIDANCE

Since the 1980s, the fitness industry has boomed, stagnated, grown again, and more suppliers have entered the market (ABS, 2006b; Brabazon, 2000; Frew & McGillivray, 2005). The resulting pressure to retain and attract clients has led to several developments in the market. One response has been to diversify fitness program approaches, offering consumers many more choices, prompting one commentator to remark that the fitness industry is a 'promiscuous paradigm' (Brabazon, 2000, p. 100). Innovations are trying to tap into new groups of clientele. 'Power yoga', for example, promises to combine 'strength, sweat and spirituality' without imposing a rigid dogma; instead it guarantees to 'encourage students to take their own spiritual path' (Anonymous, 2005). A different approach developed by the New Zealand fitness chain of Les Mills (a market leader in Australia) caters for men by emphasising structure, authority and masculinity (Brabazon, 2000, pp. 97–112).

By offering a wide range of exercise methods the industry is trying to accommodate diverse and confused customer expectations. Some aspire to achieving popular media or medical portrayals of the ideal body, while others attempt to recapture their 'former glory' (Crossley, 2005). Many consumers of fitness schemes are on an onerous journey, working towards 'a mosaic of physical, emotional, economic, and aesthetic transformations' (Glassner, 1989, p. 187). That aerobics constantly develops novel forms is a structural characteristic of the modern fitness industry in general, as it constantly turns any crisis of authority and purpose into a marketing virtue.

Another response for dealing with the omnivorous yet anxious consumers of fitness has been the growth in commercial authority, most evident in the pairing of clients with personal fitness trainers (Harris & Marandi, 2002, pp. 194–200). This approach aims to overcome a central tension within the fitness industry: clients have to be attracted by a desire to become what they are not: 'fit', 'lean', 'energetic'. Having attracted those who are dissatisfied with their lot, the industry has the challenge of retaining them. This means they must balance client satisfaction, all the while making the desired endstates constantly out of reach. As Kegan and Morse have remarked: 'One can perhaps momentarily have, but can never *be*, the perfection of the other side of the glass' (Kegan & Morse, 1988, p. 170). (See also Frew & McGillivray, 2005; Sassatelli, 2001.) The resulting disappointment, dissatisfaction and burn-out are countered by the intervention of a personal trainer: a popular form of guidance according to official statistics. Between 1996 and 2001, the number of fitness instructors increased by 61 per cent to 12 364, making this the largest sport and physical recreation occupation in Australia (ABS, 2006b, p. 43).

What makes the personal trainer an authority is to a large degree the body image and level of fitness he or she presents, combined with 'scientific' assessments of the client's body and fitness (Frew & McGillivray, 2005; Philips & Drummond, 2001). Investigating the Scottish health and fitness industry, Frew and McGillivray illustrate how medical authority is ever-present, albeit indirectly. The induction to a fitness centre is regularly conducted in a medicalised way, and includes measuring blood pressure, weight, flexibility and body fat. It is common practice to place the fitness client on a scale and ask them to commit to reaching the next stage on the scale.

Paradoxically, the industry combines scientific authority based on medical models with traditions of self-determination and self-reliance that have their origins in the countercultures of the late 1960s and 1970s, which opposed scientific authority. While the industry's multifaceted history ensures broad appeal, its inherent contradictions are likely to fuel in some a sense of confusion about the best ways of getting fit. For others, however, gyms offer a secure environment in which to experience the physicality of their own and other's bodies. Moreover, personal trainers can provide a trusting relationship necessary to support the long journey to self-improvement. What strikes many gym enthusiasts, however, is the relative absence of fat bodies. It is possible that the marketing of the fitness industry has overly emphasised the body to aspire to, deterring other bodies from identifying with the industry's services. It is equally possible that gyms and other communal fitness spaces are prohibitively expensive for many; and that the do-it-yourself aerobics DVD or cable TV channel are a relatively cheap source of advice and support to become more physically active. Home-based work-outs have the added bonus of protecting fatter bodies from the self-righteous gaze of the medically approved bodies.

FROM INCIDENTAL ACTIVITY TO ELITE SPORT: THE COMMERCIALISATION OF SPORT

The experts referred to at the beginning of the chapter noted a marked shift over the second half of the 20th century from incidental to organised physical activity, although less than one third of Australian adults participated in the latter in 2002 (ABS, 2006b, p. 18). Yet while the population overall has become less active, elite sports have assumed greater importance in both the national budget and psyche. Indeed in a survey of 24 countries, Australia was one of three countries (along with New Zealand and Israel) to derive its national pride mainly from sport. The finding was observed to be not based on sporting participation rates, rather '[i]t's about participating in a set of cultural values – like a fair go, teammateship – which you don't have to activate in your own lives' (Willcox, 2006, p. 13).

The Australian Sports Commission (ASC) is the body charged with implementing the national government's sports policy, *Backing Australia's Sporting Ability: A More Active Australia*. It has two major roles: to support an effective national sports system that offers improved participation in quality sports activities; and to foster excellence in sports performances by Australians. In its 2002–03 Budget, the Commission allocated close to $34 million on the first objective and $102 million on the second: or a 3:1 ratio in favour of elite sports.

One argument suggests that elite sports are worthy of disproportionate support relative to grass-roots involvement because Australians will be inspired to emulate their sporting heroes, thereby increasing general sporting activity. Despite all the media hype associated with the build-up to the 2000 Sydney Olympics and ParaOlympics, and the 2006 Melbourne Commonwealth Games, exercise levels did not improve among Australian adults in the period 1995 to 2004–05. Indeed, the percentage of the population engaging in moderate and high levels has declined over the last decade, with only a miniscule drop in the proportion of adults classified as being sedentary (ABS, 2006a, p. 23).

Twenty years ago, concern was expressed that the '"spillover" theory of sporting excellence' does not work: '[T]here is no evidence to suggest that this "emulation" thesis does anything whatsoever to democratize cultural activities, including sporting ones. The structural barriers that impede access to leisure pursuits still remain' (McKay, 1986, p. 122). Unequal opportunities to be physically active appear to be as much about which groups receive government financial assistance, as the level of overall funding.

Government support and funding over the last decade has tended towards centralisation, with Commonwealth funding for grass-roots sports organisations being channelled by the ASC to incorporated national sporting organisations (NSOs). These NSOs represent larger participation sports such as basketball, soccer, lawn bowls. At present 68 NSOs exist, to which state and locally based organisations can become affiliated. Their public profile, their ability to present themselves and to have an influence beyond their direct membership, depends on the NSO's ability not only to access government funding but also to attract commercial sponsorship. The ASC has established The Australian Sports Foundation to assist not-for-profit groups to raise money for eligible sports projects, and it encourages corporate partnership opportunities (www.ausport.gov.au/sponsor/supporters.asp).

Before the 1970s, commercial sponsorship was confined to a few sports, but this widened and accelerated. Corporate sponsorship quickly tripled in only five years (from $50 million in 1978 to about $150 million in 1983), with organised, professional and semi-professional spectator sports as the main beneficiaries. In those five years, 15–20 per cent of funding came from the tobacco and alcohol industries (Stewart, 1986, pp. 68–69). In 2000, business sponsorship amounted to $471 million, with the largest proportion coming from the manufacturing sector (ABS, 2006b, p. 62). In 2005, two giant food manufacturers – Nestlé and Gatorade – were major corporate supporters of the ASC.

In essence, what is fuelling organised sports and elite sports alike are public–private partnerships: the types of financing arrangements that are now used to deliver large physical infrastructure projects such as roadways and energy generation. Such arrangements provide private partners with numerous opportunities to market their commercial products and to promote themselves, although no one has yet studied the health impacts of sponsorship arrangements such as those between McDonald's and Little Athletics, Coca-Cola and Soccer, or Kellogg's and the Nippers program in Surf Life Saving.

The most potent public–private partnership is between TV stations and major fields of sport, which can be worth hundreds of millions of dollars a year to codes like Australian Rules Football or Grand Prix motor racing. It is generally agreed that the advent of television in the 1950s and 1960s accelerated the commercialisation of modern sport in Australia, leading to a 'symbiotic relationship' between sport and the media (Frey & Eitzen, 1991; Jaher, 1977). Television came to Australia relatively late compared to other Western countries, but when the necessary infrastructure was put into place by the Australian government, it was with determination and speed: the aim being to allow Australians to watch the 1956 Melbourne Olympics (Hull, 1962, p. 119).

Clearly, TV has benefited from sport (particularly elite sport) even as it has created and promoted it. It has changed the rules governing sports, their duration and seasonality, clothing and equipment, and it has influenced perceptions of what 'good' sport is, whether heroic, daring or entertaining (Stewart, 1986). In an effort to make spectator sports such as Rugby League or Australian Rules Football (Australia's most popular sport in terms of attendance) appeal to a wider national and if possible international audience, sponsorship has led to the uprooting of clubs from their local origins. Local sporting ovals have been bypassed in favour of larger city or outer-suburban, purpose-built venues; and local names have been dropped in favour of generic ones as clubs try to attract a broad supporter base, which often includes moving from one city to another (for example, the South Melbourne club became the 'Swans' when it moved to Sydney).

Competing television stations have become powerful authorities on sport and physical activity. Elite sports stars not only have their heroic feats televised while wearing sponsor logos, they appear in product advertisements and are regularly interviewed on lifestyle programs where their opinions are sought on a range of issues. The fortunes of elite sportsmen and sportswomen, of TV proprietors and of large public and private corporate sponsors appear indivisible.

THE COMMERCIALISATION OF LEISURE

Television has done more than promote elite sports, it has commercialised opportunities for physical activity more generally. Recently, the Australian Bureau of Statistics reported that after fishing, holiday travel/driving for pleasure consumed more time per day than formal or informal sport, and consumed almost three times as much time as walking per day (ABS, 2006b, p. 30). As the chapter by Hinde attests, Australia is a car-reliant nation, and the mass media advertising of cars is a ubiquitous feature of the everyday. In this way, TV has a double impact on activity and energy expenditure patterns: not only is watching television the nation's most popular pursuit in terms of time allocated to recreation and leisure activities (audio/visual media comprise almost 40 per cent of adult 'free time activities') (ABS, 2006b, p. 29), this medium encourages driving for pleasure in its many infotainment and lifestyle programs.

MYRIAD ADVISORS AND COMPETING ADVICE

'Elitism' extends beyond athletes to include other experts, such as psychologists and nutritionists. As the disciplines supporting sport have become professionalised, traditional authorities on physical activity and sport in education, like the YMCA, have been transformed into, or supplanted by, new authorities and professional groups. During the 1950s, physical education in schools began shifting away from 'drilling and exercise programs' to become 'sport based' (Kirk & Macdonald, 1998, p. 8). Since then, work opportunities for physical educators outside schools have blossomed, with, for example, a 560 per cent increase in the number of outdoor adventure leaders between 1996 and 2001 (ABS, 2006b, p. 43).

The field has fragmented into diverse organisations representing the new specialists, such as Sports Medicine Australia founded in 1963[1], the Australian Society for Sports History and the Australian Society for Sport Administration, both founded in 1983[2]. This situation has led to tensions in the traditional peak association for professionals in the field of physical activity, the Australian Council for Health, Physical Education and Recreation, and the Council has 'found it increasingly difficult to represent all of those interests in a unified manner' (Kirk & Macdonald, 1998, p. 3).

Added to the numerous professional bodies are the advocacy organisations. Bodies like Bicycle Australia and the Pedestrian Council of Australia vie for government attention, often arguing very different cases in the interests of their constituents. While the number of experts advising the wider public has increased, some critical voices have asserted that commercialisation, professionalisation and elitism have had a profoundly negative impact on grass-roots sport and general activity levels (McKay, 1986).

Diet

MYRIAD ADVISORS AND CONTESTED ADVICE

The most marked, and potentially serious, instance of competing advice is addressed in the chapter by Smith, which describes the conflicting information about feeding babies and infants. The Banwell and colleagues chapter on pressured parenting also highlights how alternative styles and approaches to childrearing can have unexpected and health-damaging repercussions for children's diet and activity. Forty years ago, parents could follow the prescriptions of the sole expert of the day (most often a mother, the doctor or maternal and child health nurse); the platform of advice to parents today is extremely crowded and noisy.

Weight loss is another area in which claim and counterclaim compete for attention. In a review of the efficacy of different weight loss programs and approaches, Katz synthesised the findings of 343 studies and concluded that 'lasting weight control' involves 'achieving an energy-controlled and balanced diet along with regular physical activity'. This conclusion would strike many as entirely 'common sense', prompting them to cite the latest scientific paper, popularised in the mass media, that claims that some forms of energy control are superior to others: low glycemic index (GI), low fat, low carbohydrate, high protein diets have all vied for attention in the last decade. Yet from the Katz review of results of scientifically conducted research:

> [t]here is little or no scientific evidence to support the contentions of the most popular diets, including those based on carbohydrate restriction (for example the Atkins' diet), those based on food combination or food proportioning (for example the Zone diet), or those based on the glycemic index (for example the South Beach Diet, the GI Diet). (Katz, 2005, p. 72)

One response to being led astray by the plethora of promotional and scientific hype regarding alternative weight loss approaches is to ignore it, and to assume a position of 'lay expert': a member of the public who bases decisions on their own research. However, in the area of diet this is so daunting as to drive individuals into the embrace of what could be called 'merchants of hope'. In April 2004:

> A search on Amazon.com using the terms 'diet', 'weight loss', and 'weight control' yields bibliographies of 85 645; 96 722; and 101 099, respectively. The same terms entered into a web search on Google yield 25 900 000; 8 620 000 and 7 770 000 sites, respectively. (Katz, 2005, p. 71)

Within this context, why is it not possible for citizens and consumers to go to governments for *the* definitive guidance regarding weight loss? For more than half a century, the American Heart Association has identified obesity as a major coronary heart disease risk factor, advocating low fat and low cholesterol diets. However, the United States government has undermined its advocacy of this dietary approach by allowing food companies to take the initiative in promoting foods laying claim to nutritional benefits, all the while not regulating the amount of sugar in low fat foods or fat levels in low sugar foods. A lack of public regulation of high fat and high sugar foods in that country has been explained by the longstanding practice of United States governments promoting and subsidising its dairy, red meat and sugar sectors (Kersh & Morone, 2002). Similarly, the Common Agriculture Policy with its producer subsidies has been shown to contribute to the burden of disease in Europe (Elinder, 2005). While Australian governments do not subsidise agricultural production, government dietary guidelines and their implementation have been influenced and compromised by the lobbying efforts of particular agri-food sectors (Duff, 2004; Lawrence & Germov, 2004). Governments are happy to support nutrition education campaigns, whether sponsored by public or private interests; but they have been reluctant to regulate food advertising to children or to apply targeted and differential taxation to food pricing, despite the fact that healthier foods like fruit and vegetables can be relatively more expensive than heavily processed foods.

THE RISE OF HYBRID AUTHORITIES, THIRD-PARTY ENDORSEMENTS AND MARKET GUIDANCE

With larger supermarkets stocking 30 000 product lines, there is a lot for consumers to choose from and a lot at stake for the producer. Battling for shelf space in an increasingly crowded marketplace has motivated producers to team up with those few authority figures who retain public respect. In the case of food, this extends to receiving endorsements from large health-related NGOs such as the National Heart Foundation (NHF), the various Cancer Councils, or professional groups such as the Dietitians Association of Australia (DAA). Promotions such as the Seven-A-Day campaign run by Coles supermarket chain with DAA, and the NHF's Pick-The-Tick logo which appears on supermarket products, exemplify third-party endorsements whereby a commercial product receives the symbolic capital and virtue of the figure with which it is associated.

Australia's pre-eminent scientific body, the CSIRO, has thrown a spotlight on the practice of associating commodities and services with authority figures through the furore surrounding its best-selling book, *The CSIRO Total Wellbeing Diet*. In part, the debate concerns the fact that much of the research underpinning the diet was paid for by the Australian Dairy Corporation and Meat and Livestock Australia. In part, it is that the scientific body has leant its name to promote a diet that has only limited scientific foundations and whose basic premise is not supported by the dietary guidelines of the National Health and Medical Research Council (NHMRC), the country's chief health research authority (the diet calls for people to eat 50 per cent more meat than the NHMRC advises). One former CSIRO scientist was reported as saying that the diet's success was not due to the evidence but to the reputation of CSIRO; however, according to the scientific journal *Nature*, the CSIRO's reputation has been put at risk because of its auspicing a meat-centred diet of unproven virtue (Eccleston, 2006, p. 23).

In contrast, the Australian Institute of Sport (AIS) has escaped criticism despite enjoining dietary advice and sponsorship placements. Visitors to the AIS nutrition department's information page are invited to obtain the online booklet *A Winning Diet*, 'a Nestlé publication which was written by AIS dietitians to provide some general advice in the area of sports nutrition'.[3] Accessing the booklet links viewers to a Nestlé web page, which also offers other 'Australian Institute of Sports official cookbooks'[4] that contain product placements and are sent out compliments of Nestlé. In this way, authoritative advice and sponsorship blur in a symbiotic relationship between the nation's top sporting facility and the world's largest food company.

Tradition versus omnivorousness: Implications for weight

Thus far we have argued that there have been two major shifts in weight-related attitudes and behaviours over the last 50 years. First, single authorities and singular approaches to everyday life no longer provide the template by which modern citizens live. Second, a rejection of traditional sources of advice has opened the field to new authorities eager to resolve the anxiety that arises from navigating the choice-saturated marketplace.

While humans are natural omnivores, is it a coincidence that rapid rises in weight have occurred at a time of transitions away from traditional and bureaucratic sources of advice towards commercialised, media dominated sources? From the material assembled here and in the chapters by Smith and Banwell and colleagues, it appears that numerous, conflicting sources of advice facilitate forms of behavioural omnivorousness that encourage weight gain. While this proposition has not to date been directly examined, there are three types of evidence that support the alternative proposition: more rule-bound approaches to diet may be protective against unhealthy weight gain. We do not know whether the same argument applies to physical activity, but it does appear that nations whose citizens depend on cycling and walking are slimmer than those who are car dependent.

The first evidence set concerns repeated comparisons of weight rises in France and the United States in the last decade (Rozin, 2005; Rozin et al., 1999; Rozin et al., 2003). With its slower rise in obesity than other developed nations, France is of great interest to obesity researchers. (See the Banwell and colleagues chapter for a discussion of French children and obesity.) Rozin and colleagues have observed that France has a culinary culture marked by home cooking and social traditions; a norm of two to three meals a day; home preparation using fresh ingredients; meals eaten at table in a highly regulated ritual; and relatively little snacking. The typical pattern is reversed in the United States where: culinary conventions are underpinned by speed (both of preparation and eating); a high proportion of meals are prepared in industrial kitchens with energy-dense ingredients; around the clock grazing is common, as is the solitary and unceremonial consumption of food. Moreover, the French approach their food with confidence and pleasure, unlike Americans who view food with suspicion concerning what it may do to their health (Rozin et al., 1999).

Some observers attribute the different quantities and speed with which food is consumed in the two countries to their different perspective on the social role of food. Thus the French eat slowly and smaller portions, seeking *petits plaisirs*, while the American tendency to rush encourages disinhibited eating. What we can say with some certainty is that the rule bound, and what some argue to be the less adventurous, French palate has to date been conducive to slower weight gain than the open, experimental approach of the United States.

A second set of studies traces urban–rural differences in health status among newly industrialising countries. For countries such as India, China and Thailand, overweight is found in the big cities not in the countryside. Not only do rural areas have fewer dining out venues (including Western fast-food options), but rural inhabitants often cling to more traditional plant-based diets (Popkin, 1993). Most food experimentation is taking place among urban populations, especially the under-30 year olds cohort. Younger, better educated people continue to eat traditional dishes at family get-togethers and periodic special events, but they also embrace ready-prepared Western foods high in fat, and confectionaries and drinks high in sugar. The rules governing their diet are evaporating, unlike rural dwellers who can only consume television images of urban foods. Similarly, rural inhabitants do not have access to the range of choices to avoid incidental exercise. Cars are expensive, labour saving devices few and work requires exertion in contrast to the sedentary nature of jobs in the city.

The third body of work includes the numerous studies of how migrants' health status deteriorates over time in countries like the United States, Canada, the United Kingdom and Australia (McDonald & Kennedy, 2005; Papadaki & Scott, 2002; Powles, 2001; Sundquist & Winkleby, 2000). Now well documented, the 'healthy migrant effect' refers to the better health status of new migrants compared to the native inhabitants of the host countries. Their positive health is attributed to a more traditional diet of vegetables, legumes and less saturated fat, more physical activity and less stress. But this advantage is lost as migrants consume a more Western diet of foods high in saturated fats and sugars and take on sedentary occupations and insecure work. Depending on the social and economic circumstances of the migrant group, acculturation to the host country's dietary practices can be either a risk or a protective factor (McDonald & Kennedy, 2005). Full immersion in the new country operates as a risk factor when few of the traditional ways of life are maintained. Conversely, too little acculturation appears to induce high levels of stress and accompanying hormonal reactions that lead to central adiposity (weight gain around the waist). Groups who maintain their health advantage move with ease between the practices of their adopted country and their home country. These fortunate, bicultural groups – the Chinese are frequently cited – approach diet in a way that steers a mid-course between deference to their ethnic cuisine and total absorption in the Western, urban diet. We are beginning to see that young Chinese, whether in China or abroad, who adopt a United States-inspired diet (large servings of processed foods and sweetened drinks) are going to be much heavier than their parents. This is happening too among the native, young inhabitants of Japan and France, again suggesting that the adoption of a diet skewed towards the products of global food conglomerates should be considered a health hazard.

While in each of these sets of evidence there are findings that are highly contingent on a host of mediating factors, they do point in a similar direction. The observance of lifeways that have durable social and cultural significance, rather than a compliant observance of new ways of life, offers some protection against the rapid rise in obesity.

Conclusion

The Australian social and economic environment is replete with multiplying products and services, many of which are now available only for a fee or charge. Until recently, citizens turned to medical and other professional authorities, religious institutions and governments for advice about matters of health and wellbeing. In only a few decades the moral and rule-bound authority of parents, churches and professionals has been displaced by market-based authorities. Within a context of thousands of dietary and activity choices, consumers seek out advisors, boundaries, rules and traditions to guide their decision-making. As a result, the opportunities for firms wishing to establish themselves as consumer guides are numerous and there has been a proliferation of scientists, charismatic individuals and businesses dispensing conflicting advice about what constitutes a healthy diet and appropriate exercise.

Despite evidence-based medical government guidelines urging 150 minutes of exercise a week and the consumption of five serves of vegetables and two serves of fruit a day, half of all Australian adults undertake insufficient physical activity, about the same proportion ignore the fruit guideline and only one in ten Australians eats the recommended daily intake of vegetables. It seems that the government and its advisory bodies cannot make themselves heard above the nutritional and physical activity cacophonies to influence behaviour. In the following chapter, Friel and Broom indicate that less educated and less wealthy Australians benefit least from the free-for-all that is the marketplace of ideas described throughout this chapter.

---

1   See Sports Medicine Australia, 'History', <www.sma.org.au/about/history.asp> [accessed 8/3/2006].

2   See the Australian Society for Sports History, 'About Us', http://www.sporthistory.org/About.htm [accessed 8/3/2006]; ASSA, 'welcome', <www.assasa.asn.au/> [accessed 8/3/2006].

3   'Topics in Sport – Nutrition', <www.ausport.gov.au/info/topics/nutrition.asp> [accessed 8/3/2006].

4   'A Winning Diet', <www.nestle.com.au/Nutrition/SportsNutrition/Winning/Default.htm> [accessed 8/3/2006].

UNEQUAL SOCIETY, UNHEALTHY WEIGHT

The social distribution of obesity

Sharon Friel and Dorothy H Broom

T he focus of this book is on how the social and physical environment comes to be obesogenic (Calle et al., 1999; Choi et al., 2005; Mathers et al., 1999). Earlier chapters explore seven social trends producing an Australian society that fosters energy imbalance in the population overall. This chapter examines how the various trends are differentially embodied. We ask whether different sub-populations display distinctive levels of obesity, and if so what might account for those differences? The sub-populations have been selected because they represent the most ubiquitous dimensions of social structure, and because many measures of ill-health have been shown to be distributed along these lines.

Societies are organised and divided along several familiar dimensions, principally class, gender, age and ethnicity. In general these elements entail not simply *difference* between groups but *hierarchy* and comparative advantage or disadvantage.

In this chapter we review evidence regarding the patterned population distribution of obesity. An adequate understanding of the occurrence and impact of excess weight requires an appreciation of these patterns, which is also essential to effective policy and program responses.

We begin with a brief overview of the global distribution of overweight and obesity. The bulk of the chapter is devoted to presenting data from Australia. While we comment briefly on the prevalence of obesity by age and ethnicity, it is beyond the scope of this chapter to cover these elements in detail. Instead, the main focus is on the structural characteristics of class (presented analytically using measures of socioeconomic position) and gender, and the interaction between those two fundamental structures.

While much research on weight considers both overweight and obesity, we concentrate on obesity[1] because of its far greater significance for health. Although overweight is a significant risk factor for becoming obese, overweight itself is not as unequivocally risky to health as obesity. The final section of the chapter explores explanations for the observed social patterns in obesity.

An inequalities lens on obesity

Like most other risk factors for ill-health, excess weight tends to be more prevalent among people further down the social and economic scale, so that sectors of the population who are most disadvantaged in other respects are also more likely to be too heavy. Internationally, this description applies mainly to rich societies, and it is very different from how one would have described the situation 100 years ago when thinness tended to be associated with malnutrition and disease (particularly tuberculosis), and hence heaviness was more prevalent among the wealthy, especially wealthy men (Rosenbaum, 1988). The reversal from the historic direct relationship to the present inverse relationship happened in less than 100 years.

Looking at obesity through a 'health inequalities' lens mobilises the insights and considerable evidence developed through efforts to understand how population health in nearly all societies follows similar socioeconomic dimensions. Despite the popular focus on individual risk behaviours as the 'causes' of obesity, health inequalities research points toward something about society that is driving the increase in unhealthy weight. The unequal distribution of the more distal and intermediate drivers of obesity add health disadvantage to those groups who are already disadvantaged in terms of wealth, power and prestige.

Such inequalities are commonly presented as 'social inequalities in health', but what are the social components being referred to? We examine inequality along the axes of socioeconomic position (SEP; also referred to as socioeconomic status or SES), gender, ethnicity and age. SEP is a multidimensional concept that reflects access to social and economic resources (Galobardes et al., 2006). It refers to people's positions in the social order, stratified by resources and prestige-based indicators of economic, educational and occupational status (Krieger et al., 1997). The chance of an individual encountering health risks is strongly dependent on their social position (Power & Matthews, 1997), but no single social indicator fully explains the nature and extent of inequality in a society, nor do all indicators relate in the same way to all health outcomes (Blane, 2006; Shaw et al., 1999).

The role of SEP in producing inequalities in health is mediated by other social relations such as gender, age and ethnicity (Gordon-Larsen et al., 2003; Krieger et al., 1997). Much research internationally indicates that the various elements are each related to the patterning of obesity (Ball, Crawford, Ireland, & Hodge, 2002). Many studies concentrate on only one of these dimensions at a time, but it is important to recognise that real people are simultaneously positioned in terms of all four (and more besides). In some instances, it is the combination of a variety of social positions that warrants attention. For example, an 18-year-old working-class urban Anglo-Australian girl acts in particular ways, is engaged in certain social relationships and attracts distinct social responses because of all those elements of who she is. A comprehensive analysis (beyond the scope of this chapter) would incorporate all these elements simultaneously.

The next section of the chapter examines which population groups are more at risk of being obese.

The extent of inequalities in obesity between countries

Global levels of overweight and obesity differ substantially (see figure 1). Generally, in countries with developed economies the

FIGURE 1 Percentage of obese (BMI ≥ 30) adults per country
SOURCE International Obesity Taskforce, Australasian Society for the Study of Obesity website: www.asso.org.au/home/obesityinfo/stats/worldwide/links, accessed March 2006.

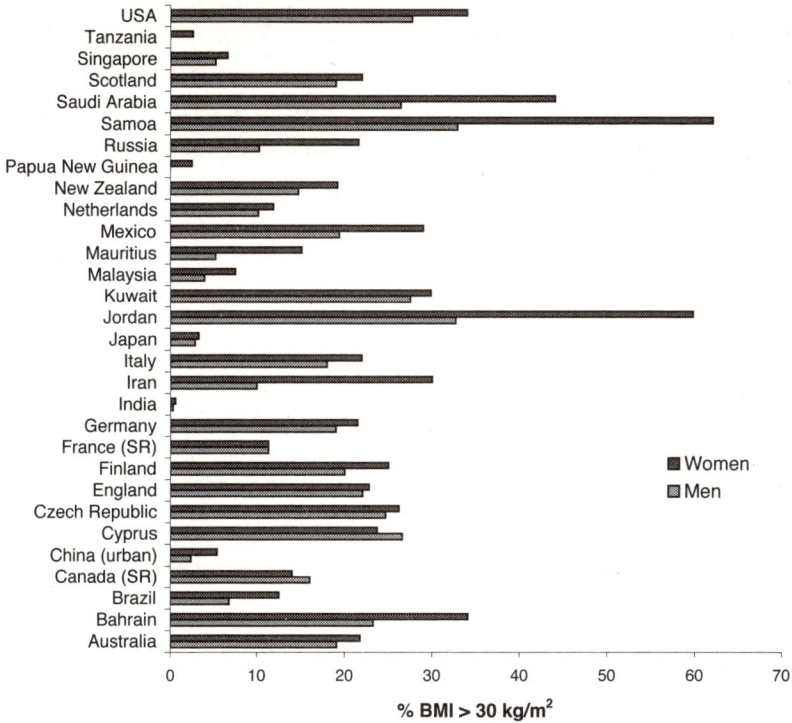

% BMI > 30 kg/m^2

prevalence of obesity is 10–15 per cent in men and 15–20 per cent in women aged 25–55 years (Seidell, 2005). In affluent societies such as Australia, the United States, and Western and Northern Europe, obesity is more common among women, older adults (65+ years) and in groups with comparatively low socioeconomic status (Seidell, 2005).

In countries with relatively low gross national product such as those in Central and Eastern Europe, Asia, Latin-America and Africa, overall rates of obesity are typically lower than in rich societies (Samoa is an exception), but the differential between the sexes is similar (Loureiro & Nayga, 2005; Seidell, 2000).

A seminal publication in 1989 (Sobal & Stunkard, 1989) reviewed the international literature, and identified a higher prevalence of obesity among more affluent men, women and children in developing societies (more like the pattern in rich societies 100 years ago). In developed economies, the review reported a strong inverse relationship between SEP and obesity among women. A recent review of international literature on developed societies (Ball & Crawford, 2005) provides reasonable evidence that the 1989 pattern of inequalities persists at the beginning of the new millennium, with persons of lower SEP being at increased risk of weight gain. In the United States, obesity is more prevalent among women with low levels of income and education, but the association is not consistent among men. Ethnic minorities are also more likely to be obese (Drewnowski & Specter, 2004). The SEP, gender and race inequalities in obesity are not confined to adults. However, the inverse relationship between SEP and obesity among white American youth is not evident among African-American or Mexican-American youth (Gordon-Larsen et al., 2003). The picture is complicated because the pattern varies depending on which indicator of SEP is used (education, occupation or income). The remainder of this chapter (focused on Australia) is informed by the need to consider obesity by different measures of social location.

The unequal distribution of obesity in Australia

The information presented here is derived from a review of publicly available data relating to population-based studies of adult obesity.[2] Surveys were identified that included measures of height, weight and one or more indicators of social difference: income, education, occupational status, age, gender and ethnic grouping. A summary of the studies' administrative details is shown in figure 12. Secondary analyses were undertaken where raw data were available. This was not always possible, and in such situations figures were compiled from published data. Unfortunately there is very little directly comparable data on obesity prevalence in different social groups over time, a problem not confined to Australia (Rosenbaum, 1988). Not every study referred to throughout the chapter contains obesity figures across all three measures of socioeconomic position, nor are they all broken down by gender. Figures 2 to 8 present obesity prevalence for Australia by gender, age, ethnic group and several measures of socioeconomic position. Note that (a) refers to self-report height and weight, (b) measured height and weight.

GENDER

In Australia as in most other nations (both developed and developing), obesity is more prevalent among women than among men. Figure 2 shows that several surveys over the last 15 years report proportionally more obese women than men in the Australian population. This occurs both when people report their own height and weight, and when it is measured by researchers. *Self-report* data from the recent National Health Survey indicate what appears to be a substantial shift in the gender difference; prevalence among men is continuing to rise (102 per cent increase between 1989 and 2005), and men now report higher levels of obesity than women. Over the same time period, the magnitude of increase for women (48 per cent) was much less than for men, although it is still very substantial in both sexes. When height and weight are *measured* objectively (see figure 3), the rapid rise in prevalence is evident, but the higher prevalence in men is not, suggesting possible gender differences in self-reporting errors (compare figures 2 and 3).

Levels of obesity in Australia show marked differences by age (see figure 4). Between 1989 and 2001, obesity increased in all age groups, but those aged 45–64 years continue to exhibit the highest prevalence among adults. More recently, however, much higher levels of obesity are being observed in younger adults than was reported previously.

SOCIOECONOMIC POSITION

As a health risk factor, we would expect obesity to be inversely related to socioeconomic position. However, the consistency of the relationship varies depending on the specific measure of SEP. The advantage of having more education is evident in figure 5, which also illustrates the marked increase in the population

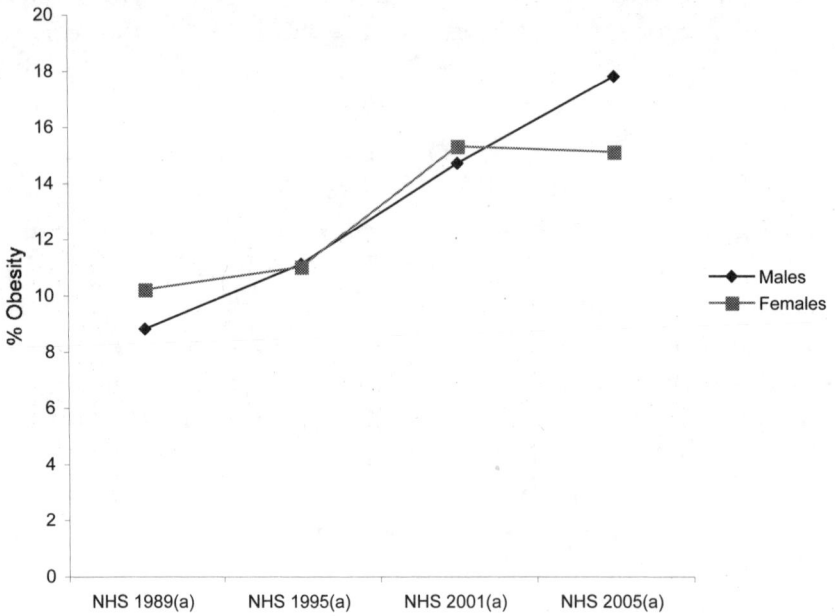

FIGURE 2 Prevalence of obesity in Australian adults by gender (1989–2005)

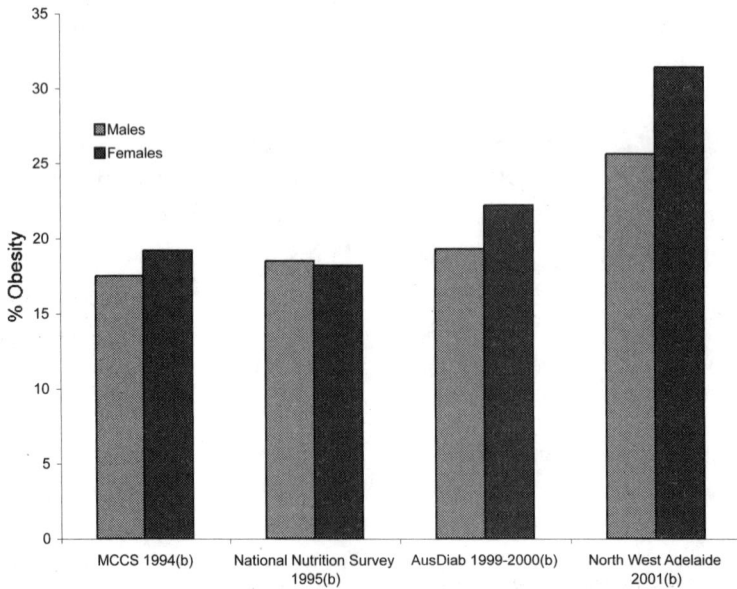

FIGURE 3 Prevalence of obesity in Australian adults by gender (1994–2001)

FIGURE 4 Prevalence of obesity in Australian adults by age category (1989–2001)

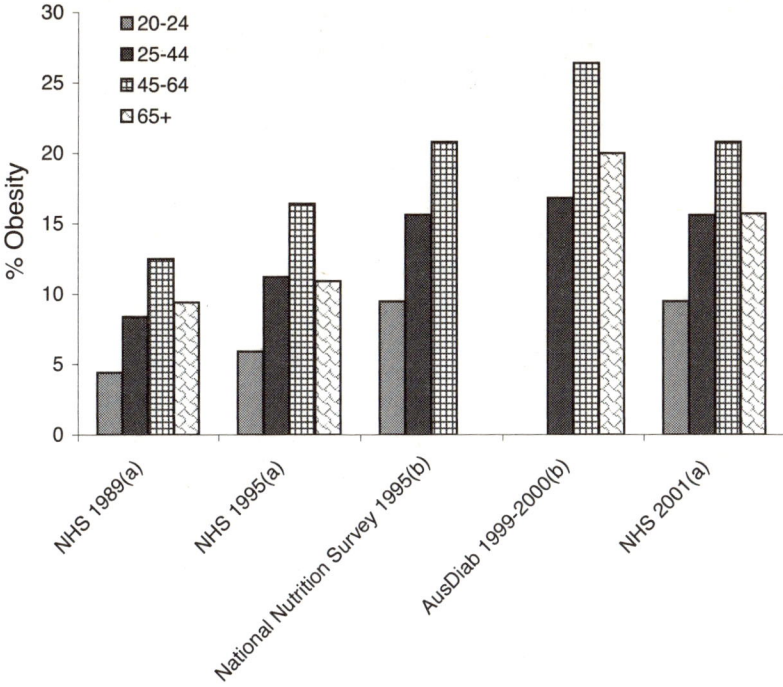

FIGURE 5 Prevalence of obesity in Australian adults by level of education (1989–2001)

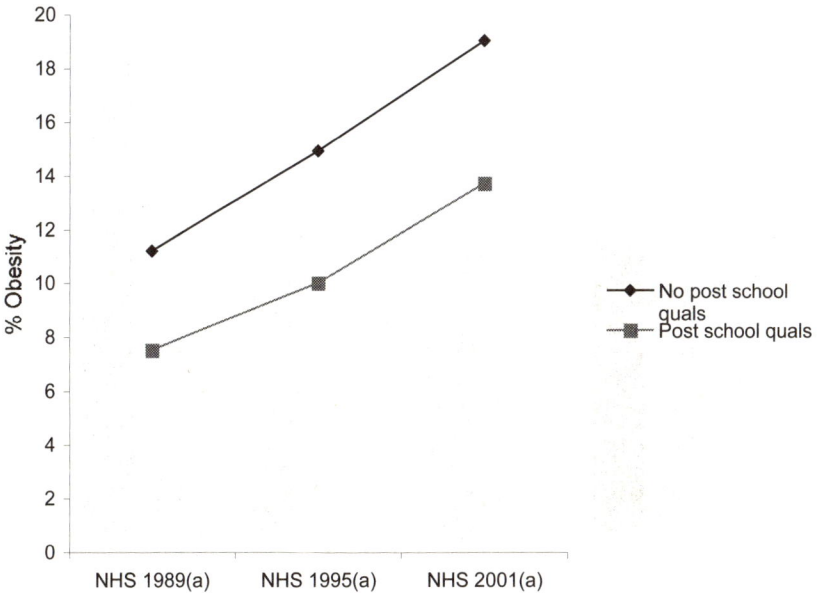

prevalence of obesity from 1989 to 2001. People with post-school qualifications were much less likely to be obese than those who lack such qualifications. Similarly, whether measured by household income, income quintile or personal weekly income, people with higher incomes are less liable to be obese than those on lower incomes (figure 6). Obesity is less prevalent among adults who are employed than among the unemployed or those not in the labour force (figure 7).

FIGURE 6 Prevalence of obesity in Australian adults by income level (Australia 1999–2001; South Australia 1991–2001)

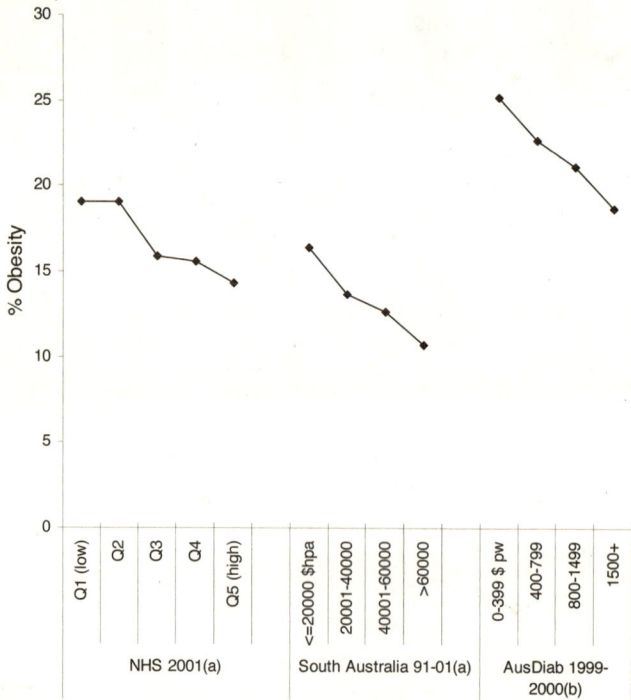

ETHNICITY

There is little national Australian data available linking ethnicity and obesity. One highly dramatic contrast can be seen in figures from the 1995 and 2001 National Health Surveys. Figure 8 shows that the prevalence of obesity is notably higher among Indigenous Australians (now nearly 30 per cent) than non-Indigenous (about 15 per cent), and it rose more steeply between the two surveys.

FIGURE 7 Prevalence of obesity in Australian adults by employment status
(1989–2001)

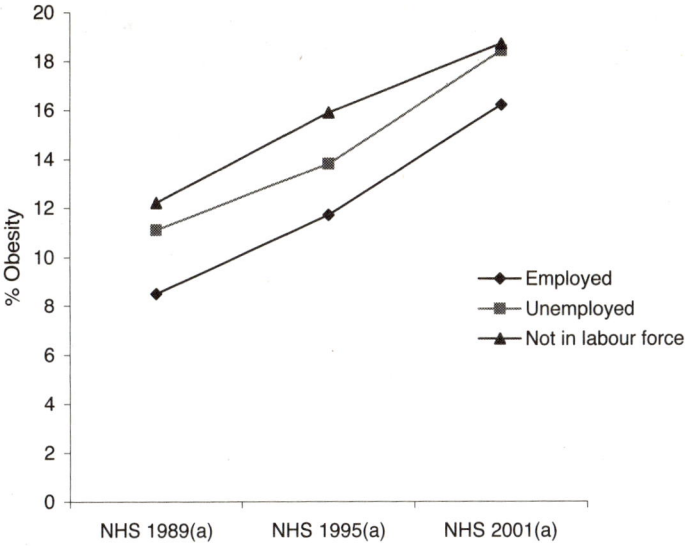

FIGURE 8 Prevalence of overweight and obesity in Australian adults by
Indigenous/non-Indigenous status (1995 and 2001)

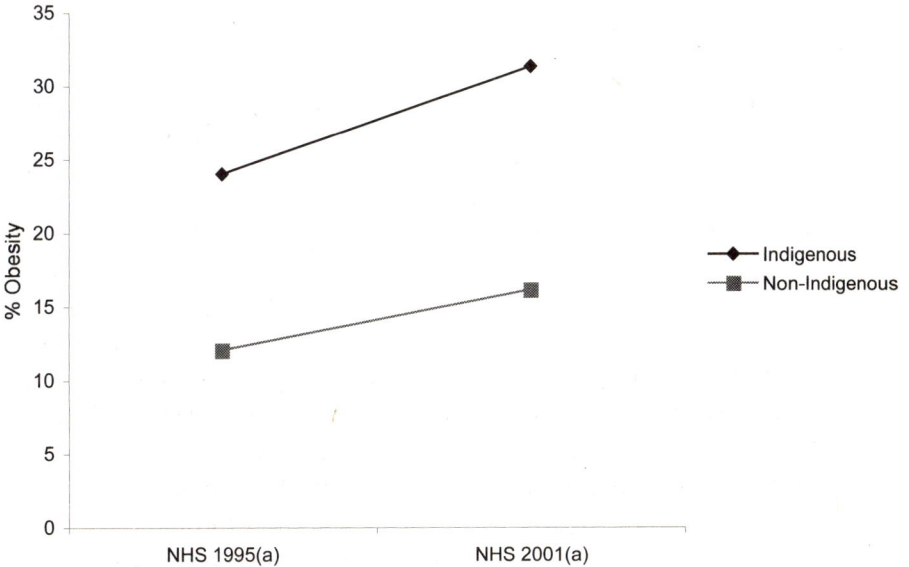

Comparisons like those in Figures 2 to 8 (which consider only one dimension of social difference at a time) cannot do justice to the complexity of social position and social relationships. Distinguishing between women and men when examining patterns of obesity and components of socioeconomic position, the picture becomes more complicated. As indicated in international research, studies from several developed nations find that the SEP pattern is relatively consistent among women but less clear or absent among men (Ball, Mishra & Crawford, 2002; Cutler et al., 2003; Eckersley, 2001; Langenberg et al., 2003; Molarius et al., 2000; Sobal & Stunkard, 1989; Wardle et al., 2002; Yu et al., 2000). Although the findings can vary depending on how both SEP and excess weight are measured (Ball & Crawford, 2005), some researchers think that the male pattern may be coming to resemble the pattern among women (Wardle & Griffith, 2001). To examine the possibility within Australia, our focus now shifts to examining (where data permits) the interaction between obesity, gender and socioeconomic position.

Figures 9 to 11 present obesity prevalence separately for men and women across the three indicators of socioeconomic position: income, occupational status and level of education. Note that (a) refers to self-report height and weight, (b) refers to measured height and weight.

Figure 9 shows the prevalence of obesity by levels of income for adult males and females. The figure suggests that the expected negative association is fairly consistent among women but is less distinct or even absent for men. Indeed, there is a suggestion of a positive relationship between obesity and income (men on higher incomes being *more* likely to be obese) in three of the studies, which is surprising because it is contrary to both the typically inverse association between SEP and health risk, and also to the pattern observed for women.

Figure 10 showing occupational ranking indicates that the anticipated inverse relationship is broadly evident for both women and men, although the middle-ranked jobs diverge from the pattern, particularly for men. Notably, occupational patterns of obesity in a workplace sample in Melbourne run contrary to

FIGURE 9 Prevalence of obesity among Australian males and females by income (Australia 1999–2000; South Australia 1991–2001, 2001; Melbourne 2003)

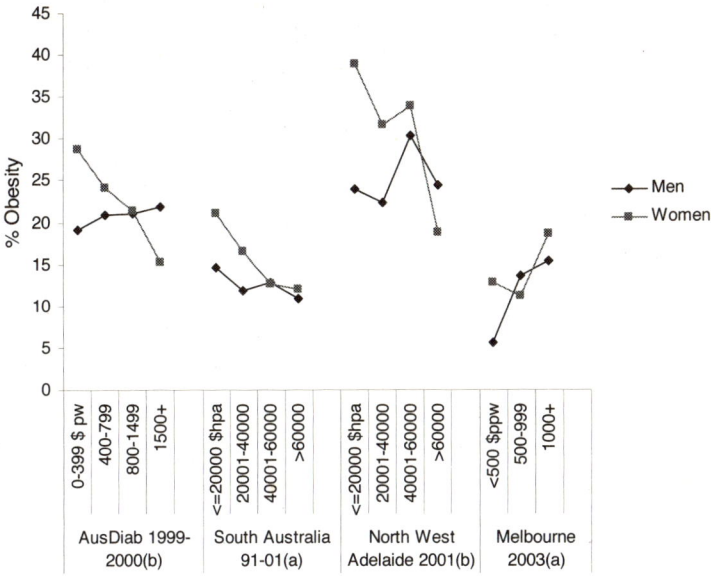

FIGURE 10 Prevalence of obesity in Australian male and female adults by occupational status (Australia 1999–2000; South Australia 1991–2001; Melbourne 2003)

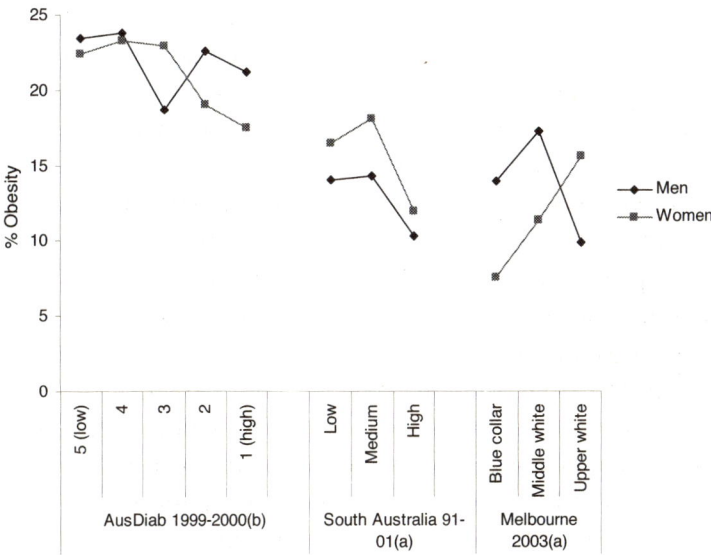

FIGURE 11 Prevalence of obesity in adults by level of education (Australia 1999–2000; South Australia 1991–2001; Melbourne 1994)

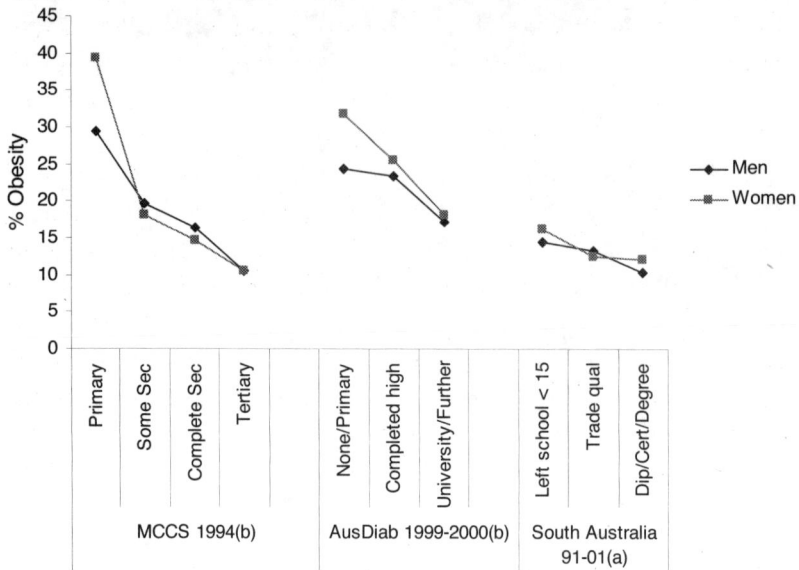

the (expected) negative relationship for women, with higher rates of obesity observed among women in upper white-collar jobs.[3]

Education presents a more consistent picture for both sexes (see figure 11) of declining prevalence of obesity with increasing amounts of education.

In summary, obesity has been unequally distributed in the Australian adult population for at least 15 years. The highest rates of obesity are found among people aged 45–64 years, and in population groups with the least education, lowest income and the unemployed. While the data show some convergence in the social patterning of obesity between men and women (as observed in some other developed nations) (Wardle & Griffith, 2001), prevalence levels may suggest that more men than women are becoming obese. Firm conclusions about a convergence or reversal are difficult to draw, however, because the nature of the relationship with obesity appears to differ for men and women, depending on the specific indicator of socioeconomic position and perhaps how obesity is assessed. Women with low education levels and low income are clearly more liable to be obese, but this inverse relationship is less consistent for occupational status. SEP indicators of inequality in obesity among men show a similar pattern to women for education, and a broadly inverse relationship for occupational status. Different to women, however, is the suggestion of a direct relationship between male obesity prevalence and income, although this is not consistent.

Of course, the diverse measures and methods used in the various surveys upon which we have drawn may have introduced systematic bias. However, three factors encourage us to think that the findings are genuine: 1) overall, the direction of inequalities in obesity prevalence is similar in most studies; 2) the consistent sex difference in obesity prevalence for most measures; and 3) the general consistency in the direction of the relationship found for each sex and indicators of SEP. These factors suggest that the observations are real patterns of inequality.

Explaining the obesity gradient

How does it come about that, overall, a greater proportion of socially disadvantaged people are obese, compared to people who are more advantaged? What causes the difference by SEP? And what might explain the gender comparisons? The question: 'What are the social factors contributing to inequalities in obesity?' leads to an extensive literature on the social determinants of inequalities in health. Although firm conclusions are difficult to draw, there are several apparent pathways involving both population-level influences and individual-level health risks (Woodward et al., 2001), so that a person's chance of becoming obese is shaped by a number of distal and intermediate factors operating, in turn, through the proximate influences of diet and physical activity.

The stratification of obesity implies that there are important structural factors involved, and necessitates consideration of the social processes underlying the unequal distribution of social conditions which promote and undermine the health of individuals and populations (Graham, 2004). Understanding the social sources of most health outcomes focuses on social position and how societal resources come to be distributed unequally between social groups. The broad sociopolitical context underpins both the societal structure and a person's position within its hierarchy. Issues of culture, class, macroeconomic policy and policies affecting labour, land, housing, education, welfare, medical care, food and sanitation establish social structures and shape the resulting form of social stratification.

But what do the social processes look like in action? How do broad population patterns of SEP and gender 'get under the skin' of women and men to shape and constrain their social identities, lifeways and social relationships so as to influence healthy weight behaviours? A start towards understanding these intricate processes can be made by returning to the example of the working class young woman mentioned at the beginning of this chapter. We'll call her Kylie.

Kylie is 18 years old and lives with her parents. Her father drives a bus for an interstate coach company, and her mother works as a receptionist for a private diagnostic imaging firm. Her father has been overweight since his thirties and became hypertensive in his mid-forties. The doctor tells him to lose weight, but he enjoys a few beers most evenings and relies on takeaway food when he is on the road. Her mother gained a few kilos with each of her three pregnancies, and is also a bit overweight. Periodically she tries new diets, mostly with little success. Occasionally Kylie's mum serves salads and stir-fry dishes, but her dad prefers pie and chips.

Kylie's two brothers are still at school, and play junior rugby during the season. She left school at 17 for a job in a discount department store where she had previously worked as a casual. Once she left school, she started paying her parents room and board, which is cheaper than getting a place of her own. The family home is in an outer suburb that is poorly served by public transport; Kylie drives to work. Although she joined a gym for a while, she is usually tired after work and she went to the gym so rarely it seemed like a waste of money so she didn't renew her membership. The store where she works is in a suburban mall, so she is constantly exposed to the sights and smells of energy-dense, low-cost fast food. When she has a night out with her girlfriends, it often involves heavy alcohol consumption. She worries about the amount of weight she has gained since she left school and started working full-time.

Several aspects of Kylie's social, economic and physical environment are obesogenic. The family's relatively low human capital is expressed in her parents and her own educational histories, which in turn limits her employment possibilities. The poor public transport infrastructure in the area where they can afford to live rules out the use of active transport options. Her parents both work in sedentary jobs, and their lack of success controlling their own weight communicates a sense of inevitable weight gain to Kylie, even though she wants to stay slim. The family is certainly not in poverty, but there is little money to spare, and a lot of Kylie's income goes on petrol for her car. Because meal breaks at work are so short, if she hasn't had time to prepare lunch before she leaves the house, it is quickest to buy a hamburger and chips. On the nights when she has to work late, she is really hungry by the time she gets off and there isn't much else open by then. It is hard for her to establish an exercise routine because her work hours change all the time.

Kylie embodies her gender and SEP. In combination with gender, the socioeconomic circumstances of her family create conditions that make a healthy weight harder to achieve and maintain. Geography, job and social relationships (both inside and outside the family) seem to conspire against her achieving healthy energy balance. Of course, Kylie and her parents are not unusual in carrying a bit of extra weight. As the population statistics (reviewed above) show, weight problems are by no means restricted to people of lower SEP or to females. Indeed, SEP and gender shape and organise the intermediary and proximal causes of obesity in complex ways. A second example is illustrative.

Like Kylie, Bruce's weight is higher than it should be – even more so: he is bordering on becoming clinically obese. In other ways, however, he couldn't be more different from her. He is a middle-aged senior corporate executive with an MBA degree, commuting in his new company car to his job in a high-rise office block in the central city where he has a reserved parking space in the basement garage. He lives with his family in an affluent inner suburb. His two adolescent children attend private schools, and his wife is a partner in a law firm. Bruce works very long days, leaving the house in the morning before the children have gone to school, staying at the office most nights until after 7 pm, and often bringing files home with him, working in his study until after midnight. There usually isn't time for breakfast in the morning, so he just grabs a cup of coffee on his way out. Except on Sundays, most lunches and dinners are eaten with clients or colleagues and include pre-meal drinks and fine wine at upmarket restaurants. He travels frequently so he spends a lot of time on planes and staying in hotels. Frequently, meals are interrupted by his mobile phone, making it hard for him to pay attention to what or how much he is eating, but he has always enjoyed his food and feels that because he works hard and earns a lot, he is entitled to eat and drink what he likes. His only exercise is a round of golf with clients on weekends (with lunch and a few beers in the clubhouse afterwards).

Despite her own professional job, Bruce's wife manages the household and children single-handed. Bruce's wife prepares the family meals, and pays attention to the latest information about healthy eating. Because Bruce eats at home so rarely, his diet is actually quite different from theirs. Although she is not a 'trophy wife', she has maintained her young adult (slim) weight while Bruce has gradually become heavier over the years. Their children might well quote the line from the song, 'Summertime': 'Your Daddy is rich, and your Mamma's good-looking.'

Bruce and Kylie illustrate how the components of SEP drive and structure the environmental and behavioural causes of obesity. And Bruce's family shows that people in one household occupying the same geographic and socioeconomic location are not necessarily affected by their location in the same ways. Class-specific gender norms, coupled with job demands, mean that Bruce and his wife experience overlapping but not identical environments, and they embody their environments in very different ways.

Synthesising the narratives and trends

Despite the fact that income, occupational status and education are correlated with one another, the various measures of SEP may generate somewhat different patterns in the distribution of obesity because they entail different resources affecting weight-related behaviour in different ways. Furthermore, the association between SEP and weight is inherently complex. For example, while high SEP is usually health protective, very long work hours (like Bruce's) may partly undermine the status advantage. There is empirical evidence that working overtime and the amount of work time spent seated are associated with excess weight (Mummery et al., 2005; Lallukka et al., 2005; Proper et al., 2006) Although high status typically entails working long hours, long hours on the job give no guarantee of achieving high status. Thus, people in lower status jobs requiring long hours (like Kylie and her father) have the worst of both worlds, and may be particularly vulnerable to obesity (Burton & Phipps, 2004). Five main points summarise the complicated interplay between SEP and obesity:

- In countries or time periods when the available food is insufficient to nourish the entire population adequately, body weight is typically positively associated with class, and working class and poor people are liable to be undernourished. This tendency is intensified where some work (paid and unpaid) requires arduous physical labour, while more wealthy portions of the population can afford servants and labour saving devices (such as the automobile) that diminish their energy output. When food becomes superabundant, and mechanisation is widespread, obesity may replace the earlier class advantage of being buffered from strenuous work and undernutrition. Thus, early in the 20th century, anxieties began to be expressed in Britain about the problem of obesity among middle-class businessmen, and both popular and medical writing addressed to these men urged moderation in eating and the development of an exercise culture designed to foster a vigorous and disciplined form of masculinity (Zweiniger-Bargielowska, 2005).

- Income is arguably the best single indicator of material living standards (Galobardes et al., 2006). As a measure of material resources, it signals the amount of money available to purchase such things as food, transport, services and leisure (Wardle et al., 2002). While energy expenditure theoretically costs nothing, in contemporary society there are often financial costs associated with physical activity (see the Banwell and colleagues chapter, this volume). And energy intake certainly does cost money. How much money an individual or household allocates to food is driven by the food available to buy, the cost of food, the resources (including time, transport, information and values) people have for purchase, storage, preparation and consumption of food (Dowler, 1997; Friel et al., 2005; Friel et al., in press; Morris et al., 2000; Rychetnik et al., 2003). In 1990–91, sufficient energy and all the nutrients (except thiamine and calcium) were available to meet nutritional needs of all Australians (Australian Bureau of Statistics, 2000). However, the marketplace is becoming more crowded with energy-dense, nutrient-empty foods, making the consumption of excess energy much easier, so that between 1985 and 1995 there was a 10 per cent increase in per capita mean intake of energy.

- Income is also an indicator of ability to purchase health-enhancing goods such as organised physical activity in the form of gym membership, foodstuffs marketed as health promoting (generally more expensive), and more expensive alcohol such as wine, which is less energy dense than many alternatives.

- Occupational status varies in prestige, and also in the extent to which employees can schedule work, develop and use skills, derive a sense of reward from their job, and receive encouragement and support to combine paid work with a healthy lifestyle. High status occupations may foster shared health beliefs and knowledge among employees, while such aspects of organisational culture may be very different in lower status jobs. Furthermore, the freedom of employees to interact and support one another is liable to be more limited where there is comparatively little autonomy and job control. For example, communication among employees at call centres is likely to be very restricted. Thus, sharing useful information and social support is highly constrained in such workplaces.

- Education is traditionally understood as a mechanism affecting health, in accord with assumptions that health behaviour arises un-problematically from health information. Level of education is known to be associated with the acquisition of health beliefs and knowledge, often referred to as cultural capital (Galobardes et al., 2006; Manor et al., 1997).

SEP through gender

Offer has asserted that the influence of class on weight occurs *through gender*. He claims that 'women's weight is more strongly determined by socioeconomic status than men's and women also care more about it' (Offer, 1998). Certainly, the Australian data presented above partly confirm the claim. If it is correct that women's weight is more strongly determined by their status,

women would be wise to 'care more about it'. Whether (
is right or not, his observation alerts us to the awkward rea
that neither SEP nor body weight can be fully understood .
reductionist terms, nor – we add – can gender.

There is indirect evidence for the logic of the class-through-gender argument. Internationally, longitudinal studies suggest that obese women incur much more significant economic penalties for their weight than obese men do, whether the penalty is measured in terms of income (Mitra, 2001) or wealth (Zagorsky, 2005). In United States research, obese white women are most disadvantaged financially by their weight, whereas white men and black women who are obese suffer comparatively limited economic disadvantage, while obese black men pay no penalty at all (Chang & Lauderdale, 2005; Zagorsky, 2005). These findings show how race, class and gender interact to complicate the interplay between weight and class, and they indicate that violating the norm of slenderness is particularly salient for women, and most salient for those women who might compete for relatively high-paying jobs, or who might marry men with such jobs.

These observations accord with women's intense interest in diets and weight control, and with men's comparative indifference or resistance to organised weight loss activities. They may also help to account for the puzzling possibility of a flat or even direct association between SEP and obesity among men but an inverse association among women. If high incomes enable the consumption of an excess of food, and demanding but sedentary jobs obstruct physical activity, higher class may become a risk factor for unhealthy weight, particularly among upper-class men who may not pay such a high penalty as upper-class women for being too heavy. While there has been a substantial shift from the more physically demanding manufacturing to service industry, perhaps men's blue collar jobs still entail enough physical activity to reduce their risk of obesity, compared to white collar jobs and working-class women's jobs. There are conflicting findings on this point (Mummery et al., 2005; Salmon Owen et al., 2000). Such important questions require extensive investigation, but we are not aware of any conclusive studies that resolve them.

Summary and conclusions

Are the patterns of social inequality in obesity we describe a true reflection of Australian society? In studies of other societies, researchers have encountered similar difficulties locating comparable data that has been rigorously collected, yet their findings reinforce the conclusion that indeed social inequality in obesity existed in the past and continues to the present day. Even with the limitation of using published group characteristics from a number of different surveys, such approaches have been used internationally to identify inequalities and temporal changes in obesity levels.

We have demonstrated the existence of inequality in the rates of obesity and argued that the inequalities in risks for unhealthy weight are economic and socially based. Recognising that the social patterning of obesity has a variety of influences, at both the individual and population level, is important conceptually and also as a basis for improving population health. One reason for identifying patterns of obesity between and within societies is to identify groups at risk and generate hypotheses concerning the underlying causes of those patterns. Not only does such information contribute to the evidence base aimed at understanding how inequalities in obesity arise, equally importantly it provides a basis on which to initiate action designed to prevent further escalation in unhealthy weight, and to redress the existing problem.

The challenge is to identify the circumstances that promote equal opportunity for successful maintenance of healthy weight and prevention of unhealthy weight, by all groups in society. The stories of Kylie and Bruce highlight the importance of equitably supportive living environments for healthy weight. Material security, a built habitat which lends itself towards easy uptake of healthier food options and participation in both organised and unorganised physical activity, a family and work environment which positively reinforces healthy living and empowers all individuals to make healthy choices, and a social network which encourages people to feel good about themselves, together build the complex web of determinants of equitable healthy weight.

A progressive approach to making each of these supportive factors a possibility among all groups in society is clearly not the responsibility of any one sector or person. A concerted response requires policies that provide the mandate to redress the systemic social, political and economic arrangements that lead to marked social inequities, which directly contribute to some groups being more at risk of obesity. It requires policies which provide infrastructures that facilitate availability of and access to healthy ways of living. It requires community-led, policy-supported action that seeks to empower individuals and societies through activities which develop social capital plus use informed, targeted education in various settings. Continuing the strong emphasis on individual responsibility through educational interventions and mass campaigns is likely to perpetuate or even exacerbate inequalities in obesity.

1   body mass index (BMI) ≥ 30 kgm².

2   At the time of writing, only preliminary prevalence estimates of obesity by gender are available from the 2005 National Health Survey. The newly released age-standardised analysis of the 1989 to 2000 Australian National Health Surveys confirms the social patterning of obesity reported here (Turrell et al., 2006).

3   The analysis of the Melbourne workplace sample was controlled for education, which may affect the findings.

FIGURE 12 Description of Australian Studies for which data is available

Study Name	Year of Collection	Collection Unit	Location	Study Design	Sample N (% Resp.)	Sample Characteristics	BMI Measure
National Health Survey (NHS)	1989	Individuals	National	X		Aged 18 +	Self-report height and weight
National Health Survey (NHS)	1995	Individuals	National	X		Aged 18 +	Self-report height and weight
National Health Survey (NHS)	2001	Individuals	National	X		Aged 18 +	Self-report height and weight
National Health Survey (NHS)	2005	Individuals	National	X		Aged 18 +	Self-report height and weight
Melbourne (Job Stress and Health Behaviours Survey)	2003	Individuals	Victoria	X	1101 (70)	Men & women In paid work Aged 18 +	Self-report height and weight
South Australia Health Omnibus Survey	1991–1998, 2001	Individuals	South Australia	X	Approx. 70 per cent	General Pop. Aged 15+	Self-report height and weight
North West Adelaide survey	2001	Individuals	West and North Adelaide	L	2523 (51)	General Pop. Aged 18+	Measured height and weight
Melbourne Collaborative Cohort Study (MCCS)	1994	Individuals	Melbourne metropolitan	L	29#799	General Pop. Aged 35–69	Measured height and weight
National Nutrition survey	1995	Individuals				General Pop.	Measured height and weight
Australian Diabetes, Obesity and Lifestyle Study (AusDiab)	1999–2000	Individuals	National	X	11#247 (55)	General Pop. Men and women Aged 25 +	Measured height and weight

X = Cross-sectional   L = Longitudinal

METHODOLOGICAL CONSIDERATIONS:

A combination of purpose and practicality shapes the methods and measures used in population surveys. Comparing data from independently designed and implemented surveys has both advantages and limitations. The most significant advantage is that findings consistent across surveys are likely to represent real phenomena, not spurious or biased results (Booth et al., 2003). However, surveys that are not specifically designed for comparison purposes, with differing methods, may contain a range of errors inherent to each method and should be taken into account when forming conclusions (Haraldsdottir, 1991). Social and economic inclusion in a survey is partly determined by the sample frame and mode of data collection (Turrell & Najman, 1995). The sample frames were not identical across surveys and the contextual interpretation of socioeconomic and demographic characteristics might have changed (Beer-Borst et al., 2000). Different survey methods may elicit different levels of response (Turrell, Patterson, Oldenburg, Gould & Roy, 2002) (Dengler R, Roberts H & Rushton L, 1997). Although all of the studies we report here used methods of random selection and had adequate response rates, it is unclear from the published documentation relating to each survey the extent to which non participation by different social groups took place. Generally, the purpose of undertaking the reported surveys differed, with the result that SEP indicators and the cut off points used to define categories are not standardised. However, the surveys did use either identical, or at least comparable, methods of measurement of height and weight, within the distinct categories of self-report or measured.

CONCLUSION

Multiple sins, multiple saviours

*Jane Dixon and Dorothy H Broom, with
input from chapter contributors*

The preceding chapters give detailed treatments of seven social environmental determinants of population weight gain. Each chapter on its own describes a complex web of causality, and demonstrates that there is no single villain behind this increasing threat to population health. Taken together, they show how the drivers of obesity are linked to one another and embedded in the fabric of daily life.

As countries modernise, their capacity to produce consumables of both positive and dubious merit increases: the cheap car, convenience food laden with sugars and saturated fats, and labour saving devices such as the remote control for the TV and garage door. But it is not simply the production of modern commodities that contributes to poor health outcomes; what counts is how consumers use them. In the language of sociology, social practices matter. A social practice is more than a behaviour: it is a cluster of related, value-laden, socially influenced behaviours. Shopping, for instance, is more complex than paying someone for goods. It involves an interplay of actions and culturally infused decisions, including decisions about how to travel to the shop; agreements as to where and when shopping should take place;

and an understanding as to what emotions are appropriate when shopping. How shoppers address these questions is influenced by features over which they have limited control or choice, namely their social status and socially informed assumptions about appropriate ways of doing things.

There are clear health risks from everyday social practices, such as using the car for every trip, using the ride-on mower when the electric or push mower would do the job, regularly purchasing convenience foods to make time to go to the gym. But the consequences are often many years away and it would seem perverse for individuals to repudiate the comforts of modernity.

Despite the richness of the information contained in this book about how unhealthy weight is socially produced, we do not claim to be comprehensive. There are other environmental determinants not discussed here (such as urban planning and design), and the ones that are included could be treated in much more detail, if space permitted. However, the task of understanding the social and economic trends underlying the dramatic population level increase in weight has been made much more difficult by lack of relevant longitudinal data, compounded by inconsistencies in measurement and continuing debate about the most accurate indicator of what counts as unhealthy weight.

Even so, a central message from the chapters is that a number of social, cultural and economic changes mean that healthy weight choices have become difficult choices. A lifestyle conducive to maintaining weight has moved farther and farther from the sphere of influence occupied by most citizens of modern Australia. That is, a number of related (but uncoordinated) incremental changes have gradually constrained personal agency as far as a lifestyle conducive to healthy weight is concerned. Individuals are not completely helpless, but the capacity to act on one's own to prevent or reverse weight gain has become limited by the nature of paid work, the design of cities, contemporary commodities and markets, and social norms surrounding gender and parental roles.

But if it is difficult to unpack and document conclusively the environmental causes of obesity, it is harder still to devise appropriate solutions. We began this book by noting the ongoing political and media debate about whether the blame for rising obesity lies with individuals or with governments and institutions. What the chapter contributors signal is that 'who is to blame?' is the wrong question. The focus belongs on understanding obesogenic social forces, and identifying practical, effective ways to modify those conditions. Given the nature of the problem, it is our view that appropriate environmental solutions will require a constructive convergence between a mobilised civil society, an enabling state and socially responsible commercial corporations.

Given the complexity of the obesogenic environment, it is not surprising that simple solutions have failed to halt the problem. For example, health promotion campaigns that concentrate on a single change in personal behaviour (such as 'eat more fruit') are too limited and fragmented to make much difference. Furthermore, such campaigns have a tendency to exacerbate the disadvantage of sections of the population already disadvantaged by low income, bad jobs and limited education. That is, the main people to take up the messages of such campaigns are those who may need them least.

But whatever individuals may want to do, the actions of large corporations, governments and international organisations such as the World Trade Organization can significantly enable or constrain the actions of individuals. For example, by some estimates, the United States government's agricultural policy subsidising the production of high fructose corn syrup (a key ingredient in sweetened drinks, and a hidden component of many products not usually thought of as highly sweetened) is making a substantial contribution to rising obesity, since it is cheap to produce and heavily promoted. The globalisation of international trade has exported the American addiction to this product, distributing it to other rich countries as well as to nations with much lower average incomes, contributing to the poignant juxtaposition of hunger and excessive nutrition (Hawkes, 2006; Sobal, 2001).

The ethics of weight

Obesity is not simply a health problem: the socioeconomic patterning of obesity is an issue of injustice, with implications for remedial and preventive policies and other actions across a range of fields (Ball & Crawford, 2005). This book demonstrates the existence of inequality in the rates of obesity (outcomes) and argues that the inequalities in risks (causes) for unhealthy weight are based in economics, culture and social hierarchies.

Social epidemiologists are beginning to document a pattern in the way modern trends give rise to health inequalities (Mackenbach, 2006): new commodities and social practices are adopted first by the affluent and powerful before moving as a social contagion to affect rich and poor alike. After some time, advantaged groups, who have greater opportunities structured into their physical and social environments, begin to spurn the more health depleting aspects of the trends, thereby establishing a cycle of inequity (Dixon et al., 2006).

The production of salutogenic environments, however, is likely to take time. Meanwhile, individuals and families will need to take action on their own account. No reader needs another exhortation to improve their personal energy balance by reducing calorie intake and increasing energy output. But many commercial weight loss schemes, products and books are for sale to tell people what they already know: that weight loss requires eating less (or differently), exercising more, or both. Although few commercial weight loss schemes can demonstrate long-term results (Tsai & Wadden, 2005), at least some of them have the potential to assist people to become more aware of obesogenic habits that are likely to have developed invisibly over many years (Crossley, 2004). Most people who are heavier than they would prefer are keenly aware that it is much easier to acquire unwanted weight than to lose it.

In this context, the types of preventive approaches that are appropriate for the whole population are not the same as those required to moderate the heightened risk of obesity among specific groups. An equity-focused response to obesity prevention recognises the need to redress the unequal distribution of opportunity to be healthy, and typically focuses attention on the relief of poverty, improving access to education and jobs, as well as raising opportunities for social support. A concerted approach to preventing disempowered, disadvantaged groups from being more at risk of obesity requires simultaneously reducing macrosocial inequality through policy initiatives, providing infrastructures that facilitate healthy ways of living, and enhancing the capacity and resilience of targeted individuals and communities through information, skills development and social capital building (Holtgrave & Crosby, 2006).

Along with other modern non-communicable diseases, obesity is often termed a 'disease of affluence'. While the metaphor is apt in that weight gain is most pronounced in times of plenty, it is misleading when one considers the graphs contained in the previous chapter. Our view is that the majority of modern diseases, like most infectious diseases before them, are 'diseases of inequality'. They disproportionately afflict the vulnerable and poor. This label calls attention to the political difficulties of tackling them.

Modifying obesogenic environments

Numerous reviews identify the most effective approaches to reduce population levels of obesity (Centers for Disease Control and Prevention, 2005; National Board of Health, 2003; National Heart Foundation of Australia, 2003; Raine, 2004; Swinburn et al., 2005; World Health Organization, 2000). In summarising a wealth of published literature, Kumaniyika and colleagues (2002) suggest that the public health community knows what needs to be done to support a change in the environmental determinants of obesogenic eating and physical activity patterns. Indeed, the causal web of influences on obesity prevalence, developed by the International Obesity Taskforce (www.iotf.org) clearly highlights the consensus surrounding the multiple factors that shape individual food intake and physical activity.

Rather than reiterating the contents of existing reviews, we describe an environmental change strategy comprised of four complementary actions required to move modern societies off the conveyor belt of rising obesity. The proposed actions focus on preventing further escalation of obesity, but they do not deal with the many issues surrounding the treatment of people who are already obese.

Earlier we used the phrase 'the enabling state' as shorthand to describe a form of government that enacts the roles of guide to the people, arbitrator of competing interests, and the institution responsible for social inclusion. For much of the 20th century, governments in OECD countries have played these roles. However, through the consolidation and expansion of the global economy, market players have begun to dominate as health and lifestyle authorities while demanding an end to bureaucratic oversight (see chapters by Dixon and Winter, and Smith). Other chapters in this volume refer to the process of 'displacements' to encapsulate subtle shifts in emphasis. There is little doubt that the Welfare State with all of its problems has been displaced by the Consumer Society with a new suite of problems (Clarke, 2004), one of which is the rapid supersizing of the people.

We do not argue that governments in Australia have been silent on weight. The 1997 National Health and Medical Research Council (NHMRC) plan – *Acting on Australia's Weight: A Strategic Plan for the Prevention of Overweight and Obesity* – contained multiple strategies targeting children and young people: inclusion of physical activity in school programs; provision of opportunities for incidental activities through improved local government planning; encouraging food providers (both public, including hospitals and schools, and private, including childcare centres) to ensure healthy food choices are available (National Health and Medical Research Centre, 1997). The National Obesity Taskforce established by the Australian government in 2003 issued *Healthy Weight 2008*, a national action agenda for children, young people and their families. All states and territories have comparable documents.

However, as our chapter authors note, national government rhetoric is undermining its own strategy documents. In justifying its refusal to regulate food advertising to children, for instance, ministers are telling parents that they alone are responsible for their own and their children's weight even though the policies emphasise the contribution of societal as well as individual determinants of obesity.

Having identified the common elements necessary to move personal and individual-level issues onto the political agenda, Kersh and Morone (2002) contend that many more years of activism by communities and scientists is required before obesity-related political action will be forthcoming. According to their analysis, tackling the smoking epidemic was simple in comparison: there was an unambiguous 'demon' commodity and industry. Further, unlike smoking everyone has to eat, and numerous industries are involved in food production and distribution. Perhaps the biggest obstacle to political action was foreshadowed in the chapter by Denniss: it appears that at this stage, national governments think their economies are gaining more in gross domestic product through unconstrained consumption, including providing goods and services for people concerned about their weight, than they are losing through healthcare costs and economic productivity lost due to a sick workforce.

The message contained in this book for all levels of government is that the human, health and economic costs to society and individuals of increased population rates of obesity cannot be blamed on the habits of individuals. Interventions need to emphasise prevention at a population level rather than concentrate on treating individuals. Unhealthy weight is a problem of the body politic rather than a problem only of individual bodies.

APPLYING LESSONS FROM PREVIOUS PUBLIC HEALTH SUCCESSES

For some, the 'obesity epidemic' is real only insofar as it is socially constructed through a 'pot-pourri of science, morality and ideological assumptions' (Campos, 2004; Gard & Wright, 2005; Jutel, 2001). These sceptics argue that the epidemic is a creature, if not a fiction, of the public health field, and is a problem for public health more than for the general public. Because the evidence is 'incomplete', 'confused' and 'contradictory' – as several chapters in this book attest – some commentators are questioning the current obsession with the issue. We agree with those who allege that body size has been medicalised and who note the lack of consensus within the medical and political fields about the nature, aetiology and solution to the problem.

These debates raise an important question about whether obesity represents a 'crisis for public health' or a 'public health crisis'. Noting the distinction between obesity and overweight, we accept the need for caution in responding to cries of alarm targeting rising rates of overweight because the data linking ill-health to overweight in adults is unclear (Dunstan et al., 2002). Moreover, for adults activity is a better predictor of health risk than overweight (Australian Bureau of Statistics, 2006). However, the doubling of adult obesity and the trebling of childhood obesity since the 1980s are alarming trends because of compelling evidence linking adolescent and adult obesity to poorer health outcomes.

Recognising a need to distinguish between overweight and obese populations, the editors believe that obesity is a critically important problem for the Australian population and for those individuals who feel distressed by their weight. Preventing further rises in obesity is important because extreme weight gain is very difficult to reverse, with surgery the most effective treatment at this stage (Jain, 2005).

Public health has two important contributions to make to obesity prevention. First, it can continue to identify patterns of obesity between and within societies and to identify groups at risk. However, demonstration alone does not solve problems. The challenge is to identify the necessary conditions that promote equal opportunity for successful maintenance of healthy weight and prevention of unhealthy weight by all groups in society.

Second, public health can apply the lessons learned in slowing and halting previous epidemics and it can broadcast the ingredients for success. Many people assume that controlling infectious diseases like tuberculosis, smallpox and cholera came about through medical science breakthroughs such as a vaccination or lifesaving drugs. What is often ignored is the way medical researchers and practitioners worked alongside governments and citizens in the 19th and early 20th centuries to improve national diets, for example, as both a driver of economic development and a defence against disease. Together with town planners, welfare reformers and municipal socialists, epidemiologists and doctors also shaped the thinking about the basic requirements of towns and cities: decent housing, sanitation and clean water.

A century later, it is clear that some of their admonitions – such as the need for space between dwellings to remove the miasma of foul air – have had unintended consequences, like urban sprawl (Newman, 2006), which as Hinde points out (this volume) is a form of city living conducive to weight gain.

On balance, public health has much to offer especially when its efforts are made in concert with groups outside the health field. In Australia there is evidence that folk knowledge and personal observations of the harms of tobacco use drove considerable opposition to the spread of smoking in the early decades of the 20th century, long before doctors and epidemiologists developed a consistent view (Tyrell, 1999). Since then, epidemiologists have played a key role supplying the evidence of a direct causal link between smoking and lung cancer, as well as joining social activists, lawyers and victims groups to plead urgent action to stop the unfettered promotion and distribution of cigarettes.

Unravelling the substantial declines in mortality due to coronary heart disease (CHD) over the last 40 years is somewhat harder than lung cancer because CHD has multiple aetiological factors, including smoking, high cholesterol, physical inactivity and high blood pressure. Improvements in rates of heart disease since the 1960s are due mainly to declines in smoking and the lowering of cholesterol (Abelson & Taylor, 2001), although it would be erroneous to assume that medicine was wholly responsible for the lowering of cholesterol. Social histories of the Australian diet reveal that wives and mothers used the emerging medical science, contained in popular media accounts, to shift household consumption away from saturated fats to poly- and mono-unsaturated fats prior to the dramatic uptake of cholesterol lowering drugs, CHD's new 'silver bullet' (Crotty, 1995; Santich, 1995).

Less well documented are the activities of public health figures negotiating behind the scenes to encourage broader modifications to the food system. Nutrition scientist Kerin O'Dea and colleagues, for instance, worked during the 1980s with the red meat industry to produce lean meat, thereby ensuring that all consumers – rich and poor alike – had ready access to a healthier option (Sindall et al., 1994). This is a relatively rare instance of the commercial environment changing its practices, without protracted struggle between an industry, community and government.

These examples confirm a view of medical historian John Powles (2001) regarding the origins of good health in the second half of the 20th century. Powles analysed three public health successes that occurred without formal public health intervention: smoking cessation in the United States in the 1950s and 1960s, transmission of HIV among homosexuals in England in the 1980s, and the decline of Sudden Infant Death Syndrome (SIDS) in England in the 1980s. He concluded that community response to new medical knowledge promulgated in the popular media was a key factor behind behaviour change.

His argument is summarised in figure 1. Economic development (in the form of increased individual incomes and technological advances) is broadly beneficial to population health but is generally accompanied by unintended health problems for both human populations and the environment. Once these penalties have been detected, often after a sustained period in which new lifestyles have evolved around the fruits of progress, it takes concerted efforts by knowledge producers and consumers, by technology producers, and by institutions like government and medicine, to respond.

FIGURE 1 The population health improvement pathway (after Powles, 2001)

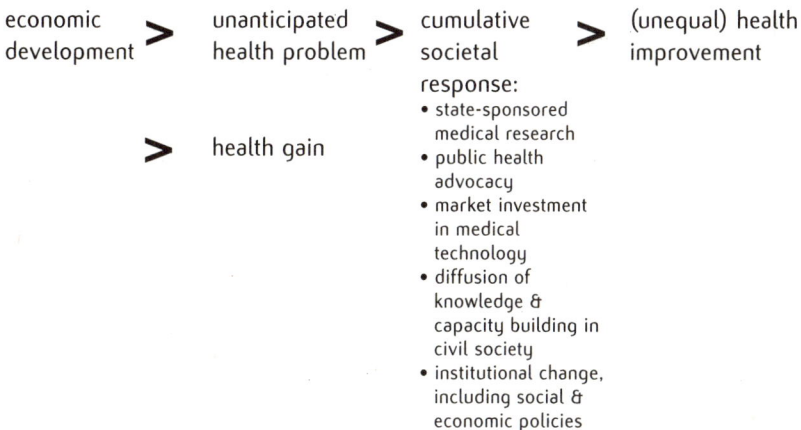

economic development > unanticipated health problem > cumulative societal response:
- state-sponsored medical research
- public health advocacy
- market investment in medical technology
- diffusion of knowledge & capacity building in civil society
- institutional change, including social & economic policies
> (unequal) health improvement

> health gain

While Powles does not dismiss the importance of what he calls 'organised efforts to protect health' – typified by government regulation of smoking, seat belts and drink-driving – he places great emphasis on the way civil society responds to new knowledge and also on the health protective and damaging role that culture may play, particularly with regard to diet.

FROM A FEEL FOR THE GAME TO A FEEL FOR THE RULES OF THE GAME

Obesity has been described as 'a cultural revolution with obvious economic roots' (Fernandez-Armesto, 2001), and in a recent review of environmental responses to the prevention of obesity, cultural factors (called 'normative attitudes') were deemed essential drivers of whether people would modify their diet and physical activity habits (Brownson et al., 2006). However, the preceding chapters indicate that groups have different normative attitudes in relation to diet and physical activity according to their social position.

The work of social scientists such as Max Weber, Pierre Bourdieu and Norbet Elias helps to explain that individuals acquire the tastes and preferences of their social group. Essentially, cultural practices as well as people's perceptions of their social status and wellbeing are seamless parts of an ongoing and unnoticed (yet socially patterned) flow of everyday existence. To explain the process that lies behind the unconscious adoption of group practices, Elias and Bourdieu used an analogy of people acquiring a 'feel for the game [of life]' through participating in ordinary and expected routines (Bourdieu, 1984; Goudsblom & Mennell, 1980). While most players accept the rules of the game, some strategically defy or set about to change the rules. Through acquiring a 'feel for the rules of the game', they are well placed to establish an alternative constellation of feelings, behaviours and routines.

It is possible to illustrate this point further by reflecting on why more advantaged groups are repudiating cheap symbols of economic progress, such as fast foods and cars, in favour of longer established ways of life, such as slow food and active transport. Dixon and Winter (this volume) debated the merits of adopting a traditional or an omnivorous approach to diet, and concluded that a more traditional diet (one less dominated by an urban, Western fast food style) appears to have protected national populations and some sub-populations against the rapid escalations of obesity. Yet we also know from Friel and Broom's analysis that upper socioeconomic groups, who are considered the more culturally adventurous (Emmison, 2003) and omnivorous (Bennett & Silva, 2006), are generally more successful at resisting weight gain. What has been largely overlooked is that omnivores value traditional ways of life as well as experimenting with the new. Socially advantaged groups practise forms of cultural rigidity as well as flexibility with regard to routines, habits and tastes (Banwell et al., 2006; Elchardus, 1991, 1994). Cultural inflexibility has even been argued to be a hallmark of privilege (Elchardus, 1994). This makes sense when one considers how affluent people are better able to control their working and living circumstances compared to those in insecure jobs and casualised labour routines, precarious rental housing markets, and the objects of constantly changing social security policies. Some can choose to be flexible when it is to their advantage while others have flexibility foisted upon them.

While holding onto culinary and physical activity traditions is becoming harder everywhere, some people are successfully navigating the obesogenic environment by using their education, social status and money (their cultural, social and economic capital in Bourdieu's terms) to modify the rules that encourage consuming the new, the convenient, the speedy and the efficient. In defying certain mass market expectations, they accumulate further cultural and economic capital as well as health capital. It is in this sense that we can talk about their having a feel for the rules of the game: they have the resources – knowledge, social connections, finances – to flout both inherited and seductively imposed conventions while creating new conventions from which they benefit. Acquiring dispositions that subvert the types of lifestyle encouraged by the seven environmental trends described in this book would go a long way to helping people to reclaim some mastery over their social circumstances.

Powles (2001) pointed out that health improvements are the result of multiple actions by multiple actors. We would add that where there is a concern for health inequalities, it is not sufficient to argue for a laissez-faire approach whereby knowledgeable and motivated individuals who change their behaviour gain the most and earlier on than other groups. Just as commercial actors constantly intervene in cultural systems through the values they project onto their products and governments shape social attitudes through the specific features and operations of their policies and programs, it is necessary to consider a more organised civil society response to cultural matters.

In practical terms, this means that everyone will need to be and feel competent to assess the risks and benefits of their various actions, and to move from largely unconscious and automated knowledge of the rules of the game to questioning the rules of the game. At various times, everyone employs what has been identified as 'lay epidemiology' to judge their health risks: that is, 'routine observation and discussion of cases of illness and death in personal networks and in the public arena' (Hunt & Emslie, 2001). As a result of what they see and experience in everyday life people form attitudes about their own health risks, ranging from viewing life as a lottery ('you never know when you'll be hit by a bus') to unqualified optimism about medical breakthroughs saving them. Useful as it is, this folk wisdom needs to be tempered by information from professional epidemiologists so that lay epidemiologists can become lay experts.

Rather than fear medical or professional hegemony in framing the understandings of obesity, we are more concerned about the consumer anxiety and 'volatile frustration' (Katz, 2005) provoked by a cacophony of competing voices and the eclipse of publicly accountable authorities. Particularly in the context of complex and obesogenic environments, governments have a duty of care to create opportunities for all citizens to acquire competence in assessing personal risks. While the 'riskiness of life won't go away' (Bauman, 2001 p. 179), citizen-consumers need to be freed as much as possible from the immobilising confusion, doubt and anxiety that accompany much popular discourse about social and health problems. More and better health education is not enough on its own. In addition, communities across the nation need ready access to publicly funded and accountable 'knowledge brokers' such as public health nutritionists and physical educators, to help interpret myriad pieces of advice and to build capacity for collective action on shared problems. This is what we mean by an organised civil society response to culture.

RECALIBRATING THE VALUE OF TIME

In discussions about giving people access to health-promoting goods and services, their cost and physical availability are usually acknowledged. We argue that access is as much about understandings of time and feelings about the pace of life as it is about money and socio-spatial arrangements. For many people, demographic and economic changes have altered how they understand the availability of time (see chapters by Broom and Strazdins, and Smith). Time pressure has become a status symbol, with successful people commonly boasting about how busy they are. We are more inclined to think that time poverty describes an emerging source of stress in contemporary societies rather than being an indication of success, and that an absence of time pressure should be counted as an indicator of quality of life (Strazdins, 2006).

Time is a precious resource, and people need time to keep healthy, to exercise, to maintain strong social bonds and to prepare nutritious meals. This is a point well recognised by producers of goods and services who have successfully convinced consumers of the value of convenience or shortcuts. Equally they have persuaded many people that leisure ('free time') is well spent consuming other people's goods and services rather than being actively engaged in their own production or in simple sociability.

In part, a consumerist orientation is justified by the efficiency inherent in the division of labour which suggests that individuals should only produce what they are expert at or at what will bring economic reward. According to one economic commentator: '[t]he problem of time's scarcity goes to the heart of the way capitalist economies are organised and the way they evolve. Indeed capital gains its value from the fact that we use it to achieve more with our time' (Gittens, 2004, p. 13). However, for many employees, recent industrial relations changes based on a flexible labour force have done little to enhance work–family balance. If employees are to feel less pressured by competing time demands, future employer–labour compacts will need to recalibrate the monetary and social value accorded to time. This includes recognition that the pattern of hours spent in employment can be as important to employee health and wellbeing as the overall number of hours on the job.

The temporal dimension to modern living is an important consideration for health promotion because many health interventions and environmental solutions have hidden time costs. Interventions such as those designed to improve walkability or use of public transport are likely to cost considerably more time than driving, especially for people whose daily travel fits in children's or elder's schedules alongside their own. The issue of time pressure poses particular problems for urban design. Time use is contoured by the way cities are designed, including transport systems, location of services, workplaces, homes, childcare and schools. If urban planning can reduce time demands (especially for those who are time poor), it may directly improve health and social outcomes. However, where planning increases time demands, it is likely to have unanticipated health costs, disadvantaging those in the community who are most time squeezed (Strazdins, 2006). If we can demonstrate that planning reduces time costs or can free up time, interventions will be more likely to succeed.

Conclusion

In the introductory chapter we noted that the rapid rise in obesity began in the 1980s in Australia, and a similar fate is befalling newly industrialising countries 20 years later. There is no definitive research to explain why the tipping point was around 25 years ago, although a plausible explanation involves the global transmission and coalescence of the seven social environmental trends described in this book. If that is accurate, debating whether individuals or societies are to blame for obesity is a distraction from constructive action.

The march of the health consequences of the seven deadly environmental sins will only be arrested if there are multiple, synergistic actions by numerous actors. Governments will need to regulate some business activities, develop unambiguous evidence-based behavioural guidelines (instead of vague advice such as 'eat a balanced diet') and sponsor health promotion knowledge brokers. Markets will have to withdraw dangerous commodities (in Spain, the fashion industry has established a voluntary code of conduct to limit the use of underweight models), produce healthy commodities (as in the example of the red meat industry) and desist from misleading advertising about the merits of their products. Employers' demands on labour will need to be tempered by concerns for home and community life, recognising that flexible work schedules can undermine as well as promote the ability to undertake vital care duties. Unions and communities must continue to agitate for decent working and living conditions, including health-promoting urban design. Scientists and the media will need to work differently if journalists are to become a useful vehicle for reporting scientific 'breakthroughs'. Finally, individuals cannot avoid becoming lay experts on matters of deep concern to them, including the very mundane issue of their weight.

REFERENCES

Introduction

<www.naafa.org>; <www.bella.co.nz>
<www.mori.com/polls/2004/bbc-heaven.shtml>
Banwell, C, Hinde, S, Dixon, J & Sibthorpe, B (2005). Reflections on expert consensus: a case study of the social trends contributing to obesity. *European Journal of Public Health, 15*(6), 564–68.
Bennett, S (2003). *Obesity Trends in Older Australians*. Canberra: AIHW.
Booth, M, Chey, T, Wake, M, Norton, K, Hesketh, K, Dollman, J et al. (2003). Change in the prevalence of overweight and obesity among young Australians, 1969–1997. *American Journal of Clinical Nutrition, 77*, 29–36.
Cameron, AJ, Welborn, TA, Zimmet, PZ, Dunstan, DW, Owen, N, Salmon, J et al. (2003). Overweight and obesity in Australia: the 1999–2000 Australian Diabetes, Obesity and Lifestyle Study (AusDiab). *Medical Journal of Australia, 178*(9), 427–32.
Campos, P (2004). *The Obesity Myth: Why America's Obsession with Weight is Hazardous to Your Health*. New York: Gotham Books.
Chang, V & Christakis, N (2002). Medical modelling of obesity: a transition from action to experience in a 20th century American textbook. *Sociology of Health and Illness, 24*(2), 151–77.

Chopra, M & Darnton-Hill, I (2004). Tobacco and obesity epidemics: not so different after all? *British Medical Journal, 328*(7455), 1558–60.

Cutler, D, Glaeser, E & Shapiro, J (2003). Why have Americans become more obese? *Journal of Economic Perspectives, 17,* 93–118.

Dixon, J (2002). *The Changing Chicken: Chooks, Cooks and Culinary Culture.* Sydney: UNSW Press.

Dixon, T & Waters, A-M (2003). *A Growing Problem: Trends and Patterns in Overweight and Obesity Among Adults in Australia, 1980 to 2001* (Cat No. AUS 36). Canberra: AIHW.

Ebberling, C, Pawlak, D & Ludwig, DS (2002). Childhood obesity: public-health crisis, common sense cure. *The Lancet, 360,* 473–82.

Eckersley, R (2004). *Well & Good: How We Feel and Why it Matters.* Melbourne: Text Publishing.

Egger, G & Swinburn, B (1997). An 'ecological' approach to the obesity pandemic. *British Medical Journal, 315*(7106), 477–80.

Flint, D (2003). *The Importance of Defending Freedom of Commercial Speech.* Sydney: Australian Association of National Advertisers.

French, S, Story, M & Perry, C (1995). Self-esteem and obesity in children and adolescents: a literature review. *Obesity Research, 3,* 479–90.

Frumkin, H, Frank, L & Jackson, R (2004). *Urban Sprawl and Public Health: Designing, Planning and Building for Healthy Communities.* Washington: Island Press.

Gill, T (1997). Key issues in the prevention of obesity. *British Medical Bulletin, 53,* 359–88.

Hill, A & Silver, E (1995). Fat, friendless and unhealthy: 9-year-old children's perception of body shape stereotypes. *International Journal of Obesity Related Metabolic Disorders, 19*(6), 423–30.

Humphreys, JS & Dixon, J (2004). Access and equity in Australian rural health services. In J Healy & M McKee (eds), *Accessing Healthcare: Responding to Diversity* (pp. 89–108). Oxford: Oxford University Press.

Jain, A (2004). Fighting obesity. *British Medical Journal, 328*(7452), 1327–28.

Joint WHO/FAO Expert Consultation (2003). *Diet, Nutrition and the Prevention of Chronic Diseases* (vol. 916). Geneva: World Health Organization.

Lambert, C (2004). The way we eat now. *Harvard Magazine, May–June,* 50–58, 98–99.

Leichter, HM (2003). 'Evil habits' and 'personal choices': assigning responsibility for health in the 20th century. *The Milbank Quarterly, 81*(4), 603–26.

McMichael, A (2001). *Human Frontiers, Environments and Disease.*

Cambridge: Cambridge University Press.

Magarey, A, Daniels, L & Boulton, T (2001). Prevalence of overweight and obesity in Australian children and adolescents: reassessment of 1985 and 1995 data against new standard international definitions. *Medical Journal of Australia, 174,* 561–64.

Marshall, E (2004, 7 May). Public enemy number one: tobacco or obesity? *Science, 304,* 804.

Mendez, M, Monteiro, C & Popkin, B (2005). Overweight exceeds underweight among women in most developing countries. *American Journal of Clinical Nutrition, 81,* 714–21.

Mintz, S (1994). Eating and being: what food means. In B Harriss-White (ed.), *Food: Multidisciplinary Perspectives* (pp. 102–15). Cambridge: Basil Blackwell.

National Health and Medical Research Council (2003). *Clinical Practice Guidelines for the Management of Overweight and Obesity in Adults.* Canberra: National Health and Medical Research Council.

National Obesity Taskforce (2003). *Healthy Weight 2008 – Australia's Future.* Canberra: National Obesity Taskforce.

Offer, A (2001). Body weight and self control in the United States and Britain since the 1950s. *Social History of Medicine, 14,* 79–106.

Olds, TS & Harten, NR (2001). One hundred years of growth: the evolution of height, mass, and body composition in Australian children, 1899–1999. *Human Biology, 73*(5), 727–38.

Olshansky, S (2005). A potential decline in life expectancy in the United States in the 21st century. *New England Journal of Medicine, 352,* 1138–45.

Parsons, T, Power, C, Logan, S & Summerbell, C (1999). Childhood predictors of adult obesity: a systematic review. *International Journal of Obesity 23*(Supplement 8), S1–S107.

Pearson, C (2003). Death to deniers of choice. *Weekend Australian,* p. 18.

Prentice, A & Jebb, S (1995). Obesity in Britain: gluttony or sloth. *British Medical Journal, 311,* 437–39.

Reidpath, D, Burns, C, Garrard, J, Mahoney, M & Townsend, M (2002). An ecological study of the relationship between social and environmental determinants of obesity. *Health and Place, 8,* 141–45.

Reidpath, DD, Chan, KY, Gifford, SM & Allotey, P (2005). 'He hath the French pox': stigma, social value and social exclusion. *Sociology of Health and Illness, 27*(4), 468–89.

Robinson, N & Creedy, S (2004, 21 June). Fat forcing services to supersize themselves. *The Australian,* p. 5.

Smith, J & Ingham, L (2005). Mother's milk and measures of economic output. *Feminist Economics, 11,* 41–62.

Sobal, J (1999). The size acceptance movement and the social construction of body weight. In J Sobal & D Maurer (eds), *Weighty Issues: Fatness and Thinness as Social Problems* (pp. 231–49). New York: Aldine de Gruyter.

Stearns, P (1997). *Fat history: Bodies and Beauty in the Modern West.* New York: New York University Press.

Stephenson, J, Bauman, A, Armstrong, T, Smith, B & Bellew, B (2000). *The Cost of Illness Attributable to Physical Inactivity in Australia.* Canberra: Commonwealth Department of Health and Aged Care and the Australian Sports Commission.

Swinburn, B, Egger, G & Raza, F (1999). Dissecting obesogenic environments: the development and application of a framework for identifying and prioritizing environmental interventions for obesity. *Preventive Medicine, 29*(6 Pt 1), 563–70.

Vandegrift, D & Yoked, T (2004). Obesity rates, income and suburban sprawl: an analysis of US states. *Health and Place, 10,* 221–29.

Vermeer, T (2004, 30 May). Unhealthy kids face a lifetime of obesity: Governor's warning. *Sunday Telegraph,* p. 4.

Wake, M, Salmon, L, Waters, E, Wright, M & Hesketh, K (2002). Parent-reported health status of overweight and obese Australian primary school children: a cross-sectional population survey. *International Journal of Obesity, 26,* 717–24.

Sin#1 The commodified environment

Australian Bureau of Statistics (2006). *National Income, Expenditure and Product.* (Cat. No. 5206.0). Canberra: ABS.

Australian Institute of Health and Welfare (AIHW) (2004). A rising epidemic: obesity in Australian children and adolescents. Retrieved from <www.aihw.gov.au/riskfactors/data_briefing_no_2.pdf>.

—— (AIHW) (2005). Australia's welfare 2005. Retrieved from <www.aihw.gov.au/publications/index.cfm/title/10186>.

Campos, P (2004). *The Obesity Myth: Why America's Obsession with Weight is Hazardous to Your Health.* New York: Gotham Books.

Cevero, R & Duncan, M (2003). Walking, bicycling, and urban landscapes: evidence from the San Francisco Bay area. *American Journal of Public Health, 93*(9), 1478.

Chopra, M & Darnton-Hill, I (2004). Tobacco and obesity epidemics: not so different after all? *British Medical Journal, 328*(7455), 1558–60.

Chou, S-Y, Grossman, M & Saffer, H (2004). An economic analysis of adult obesity: results from the Behavioural Risk Factor

Surveillance System. *Journal of Health Economics, 23*(3), 565–87.

Coulter, K & Coulter, R (2005). Size does matter: the effects of magnitude representation congruency on price perceptions and purchase likelihood. *Journal of Consumer Psychology, 15*(1), 64.

Cutler, D, Glaeser, E & Shapiro, J (2003). Why have Americans become more obese? *Journal of Economic Perspectives, 17*, 93–118.

DCITA (2005). *Current State of Play 2005.* Canberra: DCITA.

Denniss, R (2003). *Annual Leave in Australia: An Analysis of Entitlements, Usage and Preferences.* Canberra: The Australia Institute.

Frumkin, H, Frank, L & Jackson, R (2004). *Urban Sprawl and Public Health: Designing, Planning and Building for Healthy Communities.* Washington: Island Press.

Greenpeace (2002). Join the world with Kyoto. Retrieved from <www. greenpeace.org.au/climate/government/index.html>.

Hamilton, C (2003). *Overconsumption in Australia: The Rise of the Middle-class Battler.* Canberra: The Australia Institute.

Hayek, F (1972). *The Constitution of Liberty.* Chicago: Henry Regnery and Co.

Herzlinger, R (2002). Let's put consumers in charge of health care. *Harvard Business Review, 80*(7), 44.

Hodgson, B (2001). *Economics as a Moral Science.* Berlin: Springer-Verlag.

Lee, J (2005, 17 November). Internet the saviour despite lack of imagination. *Sydney Morning Herald,* p. 23.

Metherell, M (2006, 12 April). Junk food ban off road. *Sydney Morning Herald,* p. 4.

Pocock, B (2003). *Work Life Collision.* Annandale: Federation Press.

QSR (2006). Burger King introduces value meals. Retrieved from <www.asrmagazine.com/shells/full.phtml?i = 3278>.

Torres, L, Pina, V & Acerete, B (2006). E-governance developments in European Union cities: reshaping government's relationship with citizens. *Governance: An International Journal of Policy, 19*(2), 277–302.

Sin#2 The harried environment

Anderson, PM, Butcher, KF & Levine, PB (2003). Maternal employment and overweight children. *Journal of Health Economics, 22*(3), 477–504.

Australian Bureau of Statistics (2003). *Australian Social Trends 2003.* Canberra: ABS.

Banwell, C, Hinde, S, Dixon, J & Sibthorpe, B (2005). Reflections on expert consensus: a case study of the social trends contributing to obesity. *European Journal of Public Health, 15*(6), 564–68.

Bittman, M & Wajcman, J (2000). Rush hour: the character of leisure time and gender equity. *Social Forces, 79*(1), 165–89.

Broom, DH (1986). The occupational health of houseworkers. *Australian Feminist Studies*(2), 15–34.

—— (under review). Gendered configurations of chronic illness: femininity and masculinity in diabetes Type 2. *Sociology of Health and Illness.*

Broom, DH & Whittaker, A (2004). Controlling diabetes, controlling diabetics: moral language in the management of diabetes type 2. *Social Science and Medicine, 58*(11), 2371–82.

Brown, P & Warner-Smith, P (2005). The Taylorisation of family time: an effective strategy in the struggle to 'manage' work and life? *Annals of Leisure Research, 8*(2–3), 76–90.

Cass, N, Shove, E & Urry, J (2005). Social exclusion, mobility and access. *Sociological Review, 53*(3), 539–55.

Colman, R (1999). *Made to Measure: Gender Equity in the Genuine Progress Index.* Halifax, Nova Scotia: Maritime Centre of Excellence for Women's Health.

Craig, L & Bittman, M (2005). *The Effects of Children on Adults' Time Use: Analysis of the Incremental Time Costs of Children in Australia* (SPRC Discussion Paper No. 143). Sydney: University of New South Wales.

Dallman, MF, LaFleur, SE, Pecoraro, NC, Gomez, F, Houshyar, H & Akana, SF (2004). Minireview: glucocorticoids – food intake, abdominal obesity, and wealthy nations in 2004. *Endocrinology, 145*(6), 2633–38.

Daniel, M, O'Dea, K, Rowley, KG, McDermott, R & Kelly, S (1999). Glycated hemoglobin as an indicator of social environmental stress among Indigenous versus Westernized populations. *Preventive Medicine, 29*(5), 405–13.

Darton, D & Hurrell, K (2005). *People Working Part-time Below their Potential.* Manchester, UK: Equal Opportunities Commission.

Davison, G (1993). *The Unforgiving Minute: How Australians Learned to Tell the Time.* Melbourne: Oxford University Press.

Ehrenreich, B (2001). *Nickle and Dimed: On (Not) Getting By in America.* New York: Henry Holt and Company.

Floro, MS & Miles, M (2001). *Time Use and Overlapping Activities: Evidence from Australia* (SPRC Discussion Paper No. 112). Sydney: University of New South Wales.

Gershuny, J (2005). Busyness as the badge of honor for the new superordinate working class. *Social Research, 72*(2), 287–314.

Gleick, J (1999). *Faster: The Acceleration of Just About Everything.* London: Abacus.

Goodin, RE, Rice, JM, Bittman, M & Saunders, P (2002). *The Time-Pressure Illusion: Discretionary Time versus Free Time* (SPRC Discussion Paper No. 115). Sydney: University of New South Wales.

Greenfeld, L (2005). When the sky is the limit: busyness in contemporary American society. *Social Research, 72*(2), 315–38.

Gross, DR (1984). Time allocation: a tool for the study of cultural behavior. *Annual Review of Anthropology, 13*, 519–58.

Hamilton, C & Mail, E (2003). *Downshifting in Australia: A Sea-change in the Pursuit of Happiness (Working Paper number 50)*. Canberra: The Australia Institute.

Hochschild, AR (1997). *The Time Bind: When Work Becomes Home and Home Becomes Work*. New York: Henry Holt and Company.

International Labor Organization (1999). Working longer, working better? *World of Work, 31*(September/October), Retrieved from <www.ilo.org/public/english/bureau/inf/magazine/31/work.htm>.

Kouvonen, A, Kivimaki, M, Cox, S, Cox, T & Vahtera, J (2005). Relationship between work stress and body mass index among 45,810 female and male employees. *Psychosomatic Medicine, 67*(4), 577–83.

Lallukka, T, Laaksonen, M, Martikainen, P, Sarlio-Lahteenkorva, S & Lahelma, E (2005). Psychosocial working conditions and weight gain among employees. *29*(8), 909–15.

Leino-Arjas, P, Solovieva, S, Riihimaki, H, Kirjonen, J & Telama, R (2004). Leisure time, physical activity and strenuousness of work as predictors of physical functioning: a 28 year follow up of a cohort of industrial employees. *Occupational and Environmental Medicine, 61*(12), 1032–38.

Levine, R (2005). The geography of busyness. *Social Research, 72*(2), 355–67.

McEwen, BS (1998). Protective and damaging effects of stress mediators. *New England Journal of Medicine, 338*(3), 171–79.

Mann, L & Tan, C (1993). The hassled decision maker: the effects of perceived time pressure on information processing in decision making. *Australian Journal of Management, 18*(2), 197–210.

Marmot, M & Wilkinson, RG (eds) (1999). *Social Determinants of Health*. Oxford: Oxford University Press.

Mattingly, MJ & Bianchi, SM (2003). Gender differences in the quantity and quality of free time. *Social Forces, 81*(3), 999–1030.

Medibank Private (2005). *The Health of Australia's Workforce*. Medibank Private Limited.

Mummery, WK, Schofield, GM, Steele, R, Eakin, EG & Brown, WJ (2005). Occupational sitting time and overweight and obesity in

Australian workers. *American Journal of Preventive Medicine, 29*(2), 91–97.

Nyland, C (1986). Capitalism and the history of work-time thought. *British Journal of Sociology, 37*, 513–34.

Ostry, AS, Radi, S, Louie, AM & LaMontagne, AD (2006). Psychosocial and other working conditions in relation to body mass index in a representative sample of Australian workers. *BMC Public Health, 6*(53), doi:10.1186/1471–2458–1186–1153.

Peyrot, M, McMurry, JF & Kruger, DF (1999). A biopsychosocial model of glycemic control in diabetes: stress, coping and regimen adherence. *Journal of Health and Social Behavior, 40*(June), 141–58.

Phipps, SA, Lethbridge, L & Burton, P (forthcoming). Long-run consequences of parental paid work hours for child overweight status in Canada. *Social Science and Medicine*, in press.

Pocock, B & Clarke, J (2004). *Can't Buy Me Love? Young Australians' Views on Work, Time, Guilt and their Own Consumption* (Discussion Paper No. 61). Canberra: The Australia Institute.

Proper, KI, Cerin, E, Brown, WJ & Owen, N (2006). Sitting time and socioeconomic differences in overweight and obesity. *International Journal of Obesity, International Journal of Obesity advance online publication, 25 April 2006*, doi:10.1038/sj.ijo.0803357.

Robinson, J & Godbey, G (1999). *Time for Life: The Surprising Ways Americans Use their Time* (2nd edn). University Park: Pennsylvania State University Press.

Robinson, JP & Godbey, G (2005). Busyness as usual. *Social Research, 72*(2), 407–46.

Rosmond, R (2005). Role of stress in the pathogenesis of the metabolic syndrome. *Psychoneuroendocrinology, 30*(1), 1–10.

Salonen, JT, Slater, JS, Tuomilehto, J & Rauramaa, R (1988). Leisure time and occupational physical activity: risk of death from ischaemic heart disease. *American Journal of Epidemiology, 127*(1), 87–94.

Sayer, LC (2005). Gender, time, and inequality: trends in women's and men's paid work, unpaid work, and free time. *Social Forces, 84*(1), 285–304.

Sayer, LC & Mattingly, MJ (forthcoming). Under pressure: gender differences in the relationship between free time and feeling rushed. *Journal of Marriage and Family*, in press.

Schor, J (1992). *The Overworked American*. New York: Basic Books.

Thompson, EP (1967). Time, work-discipline and industrial capitalism. *Past and Present, 38*(1), 56–97.

Wooden, M (2001). The growth in 'unpaid' working time'. *Economic Papers, 20*(1), 29–43.

Sin#3 The pressured parenting environment

Anderson, P, Butcher, K & Levine, P (2003). Maternal employment and overweight children. *Journal of Health Economics, 22,* 477–504.

Aranda Primary School (2006). *Aranda Newsletter, 30th March.* Canberra: Aranda Primary School.

Australian Bureau of Statistics (1998). *Australian Social Trends 1998: Health Related Actions: Food and Energy Intake.* Canberra: ABS. Retrieved from <www.abs.gov.au/ausstats/abs@.nfs>.

—— (2003a). *Australian Social Trends, 2003: Family Functioning: Balancing Family and Work.* Canberra: ABS.

—— (2003b). *Sports and Recreation: A Statistical Overview.* (Cat No. 4156.0). Canberra: ABS.

Ball, K, Bauman, A & Leslie, E (2001). Perceived environmental aesthetics and convenience and company are associated with walking for exercise among Australian adults. *Preventive Medicine, 33,* 434–40.

Banwell, C (2003). Methadone mothers: converging drug and mothering discourses and identities. *Sites: A Journal of Social Anthropology and Cultural Studies, 1*(1), 133–60.

Banwell, C & Bammer, G (unpublished). Maternal habits: narratives of mothering, social position and drug-use. *International Journal of Drug Policy.*

Banwell, C, Hinde, S, Dixon, J & Sibthorpe, B (2005). Reflections on expert consensus: a case study of the social trends contributing to obesity. *European Journal of Public Health, 15,* 564–68.

Bittman, M (1999). Parenthood without penalty: time use and public policy in Australia and Finland. *Feminist Economics, 5*(3), 27–42.

Boulton, M (1983). *On Being a Mother.* London: Tavistock.

Brown, S, Small, R & Lumley, R (1997). Being a 'good mother'. *Journal of Reproductive and Infant Psychology, 15,* 185–200.

Cameron, A, Welborn, T, Zimmet, P, Dunstan, D, Owen, N, Salmon, J et al. (2003). Overweight and obesity in Australia: the 1999–2000 Australian diabetes, obesity and lifestyle study (AusDiab). *Medical Journal of Australia, 178*(9), 427–32.

Carlin, J, Stevenson, M, Roberts, I, Bennett, C, Gelman, A & Nolan, T (1997). Walking to school and traffic exposure in Australian children. *Australian and New Zealand Journal of Public Health 21,* 286–92.

Caterson, I (1999). What should we do about overweight and obesity? *Medical Journal of Australia, 171,* 599–600.

Clarke, A (2003). Maternity and materiality. In J Taylor, L Layne & D Wozniak (eds), *Consuming Motherhood.* New Brunswick, New Jersey: Rutgers University Press.

Cooke, L (2004). The development and modification of children's eating habits. *Nutrition Bulletin, 29,* 31–35.

Coveney, J (1999). The government of the table: nutrition expertise and the social organisation of family food habits. In J Germov & L Williams (eds), *A Sociology of Food and Nutrition: The Social Appetite* (pp. 259–75). Melbourne: Oxford University Press.

Dietitians Association of Australia (2003). *Dietitians Association of Australia Statement: Television Advertising of Food to Children.* Dietitians Association of Australia.

Dixon, J (2002). *The Changing Chicken: Chooks, Cooks and Culinary Culture.* Sydney: UNSW Press.

Dixon, J & Banwell, C (2004). Heading the table: parenting and the junior consumer. *British Food Journal, 106*(3) 181–93.

Fisher, J (1999). Restricting access to foods and children's eating. *Appetite, 32,* 405–19.

Gable, S & Lutz, S (2000). Household, Parent and Child Contributions to Childhood Obesity. *Family Relations, 49*(3), 293–300.

Gill, T, Rangan, A & Webb, K (2006). The weight of evidence suggests that soft drinks are a major issue in childhood and adolescent obesity. *Medical Journal of Australia, 184,* 263–64.

Gillman, M, Rifas-Shiman, S, Frazier, L, Rockett, H, Camargo, C, Field, A et al. (2000). Family dinner and diet quality among older children and adolescents. *Archives Family Medicine, 9,* 235–40.

Hays, S (1996). *The Cultural Contradictions of Motherhood.* New Haven: Yale University Press.

Kavanagh, A, Goller, J, King, T, Jolley, D, Crawford, D & Turrell, G (2005). Urban area disadvantage and physical activity: a multilevel study in Melbourne, Australia. *Journal of Epidemiology and Community Health, 59,* 934–40.

Livingstone, S & Helsper, E (2004). Advertising foods to children: understanding promotion in the context of children's daily lives. Department of Media & Communications, London School of Economics & Political Science. Retrieved 25 March 2006 from <www. ofcom.org.uk/research/tv/reports/food_ads/appendix2.pdf>.

Lupton, D (2000). 'A love/hate relationship': the ideals and experiences of first-time mothers. *Journal of Sociology, 36*(1), 50–63.

Lupton, D & Fenwick, J (2001). 'They've forgotten that I'm the mum': constructing and practising motherhood in special care nurseries. *Social Science and Medicine, 53,* 1011–21.

Mackett, R, Lucas, L, Paskins, J & Turbin, J (2005). The therapeutic value of children's everyday travel. *Transportation Research Part A, 39,* 205–19.

Magarey, A, Daniels, L, Boulton, T, Cockington, R (2003). Predicting obesity in early adulthood from childhood and parental obesity.

International Journal of Obesity, 27(4), 505–13.

Mamun, A, Lawlor, D, O'Callaghan, M, Williams, G & Najman, J (2005). Positive maternal attitude to the family eating together decreases the risk of adolescent overweight. *Obesity Research*, 13(8), 1422–30.

Marquis, M (2004). Strategies for influencing parental decisions on food purchasing. *Journal of Consumer Marketing*, 21(2), 134–43.

Miller, D (2004). How infants grow mothers. In J Taylor, L Layne & D Wozniak (eds), *Consuming Motherhood* (p. 39). New Brunswick, New Jersey: Rutgers University Press.

Nolan, N (2003). The ins and outs of skateboarding and transgression in public space in Newcastle, Australia. *Australian Geographer*, 34(3), 311–27.

Palmer, C, Ziersch, A, Arthurson, K & Baum, F (2005). 'Danger lurks round every corner': fear of crime and its impact on opportunities for social interaction in stigmatised Australian suburbs. *Urban Policy and Research*, 23(4), 393–411.

Percival, R & Harding, A (2005). *The Estimated Costs of Children in Australian Families in 2005–2006: Commissioned Research Report of the Ministerial Task Force on Child Support*. Canberra: NATSEM, University of Canberra.

Prentice, A & Jebb, S (2003). Fast foods, energy density and obesity: a possible mechanistic link. *Obesity Reviews*, 4, 187–94.

Ridge, T (2003). Listening to children: developing a child-centred approach to childhood poverty in the UK. *Family Matters*, 65(Winter), 4–9.

Salmon, J, Campbell, K & Crawford, D (2006). Television viewing habits associated with obesity risk factors: a survey of Melbourne schoolchildren. *Medical Journal of Australia*, 184(2), 64–67.

Saunders, P (1999). Budget standards and the costs of children. *Family Matters*, 53(Winter), 63–70.

Schwartz, M & Puhl, R (2003). Childhood obesity: a societal problem to solve. *Obesity Reviews*, 4, 57–71.

Sieter, E (1998). Children's desires/mothers' dilemmas. The social contexts of consumption. In H Jenkins (ed.), *The Children's Culture Reader* (pp. 297–317). New York and London: New York University Press.

Stearns, P (1999). Children and weight control. In J Sobal & D Maurer (eds), *Weighty Issues: Fatness and Thinness as Social Problems* (pp. 11–30). New York: Aldine De Gruyter.

—— (2003). *Anxious Parents: A History of Childrearing in America*. New York: New York Press.

Strauss, R & Knight, J (1999). Influence of the home environment on the development of obesity in children. *Pediatrics*, 103(6), 85–93.

Taylor, J (2004). *Life Chances: The Children's View*. Paper presented at the Critical Early Childhood Years Conference, Queen Elizabeth Centre, Melbourne.

Timperio, A, Ball, K, Salmon, J, Roberts, R, Geo, M, Giles-Corti, B et al. (2006). Personal, family, social and environmental correlates of active commuting to school. *American Journal of Preventive Medicine, 30*(1), 45–51.

Veugelers, P & Fitzgerald, A (2005). Prevalence of risk factors for childhood overweight and obesity. *Canadian Medical Association Journal, 173*(6), 607–13.

Warde, A, Shove, E & Southerton, D (1998). *Convenience, Schedules and Sustainability (draft paper for ESF workshop on sustainable consumption)*. Lancaster: Department of Sociology, Lancaster University.

Wardle, J, Cooke, L, Gibson, L, Sapochnick, M, Sheiham, A & Lawson, M (2003). Increasing children's acceptance of vegetables: a randomised trial of guidance to parents. *Appetite, 40*(2), 155–62.

Whitten, K, McCreanor, T & Kearns, R (2003). The place of neighbourhood in social cohesion: insights from Massey, West Auckland. *Urban Policy and Research, 21*(4), 321–38.

Williams, J (2000). From difference, to dominance to domesticity: care as work, gender as tradition. *Chicago-Kent Law Review, 76,* 1441–93.

Sin#4 The technological environment

Andersen, RE (2000). The spread of the childhood obesity epidemic. *Canadian Medical Association Journal, 163*(11), 1461–62.

Australian Bureau of Statistics (1997). *Sport and Recreation: A Statistical Overview, Australia, 1997*. Canberra: ABS.

——(2006). *Sport and Recreation: A Statistical Overview, Australia, 2003* (Cat. No. 4156.0). Canberra: ABS.

Australian Institute of Health and Welfare (AIHW) (2004). A rising epidemic: obesity in Australian children and adolescents. Retrieved from <www.aihw.gov.au/riskfactors/data_briefing_no_2.pdf>.

—— (2005). *A Picture of Australia's Children*. Canberra: AIHW.

Beck, U (1992). *Risk Society: Towards a New Modernity*. London: Sage.

Booth, M, Chey, T, Wake, M, Norton, K, Hesketh, K, Dollman, J et al. (2003). Change in the prevalence of overweight and obesity among young Australians, 1969–1997. *American Journal of Clinical Nutrition, 77,* 29–36.

Botero, D & Wolfsdorf, JI (2005). Diabetes Mellitus in children and adolescents. *Archives of Medical Research, 36*(3), 281–90.

Burdette, HL & Whitaker, RC (2005). A national survey of neighborhood safety, outdoor play, television viewing, and obesity in preschool children (Abstract). *Pediatrics, 116*(3), 657–62.

Butcher, M & Thomas, ME (2003). *Ingenious: Emerging Youth Cultures in Urban Australia.* Sydney: Pluto Press.

Carter, O (2005). Changes in obesity, sedentary behaviours and Perth children's television viewing from 1960 to 2003. *Australian and New Zealand Journal of Public Health, 29*(2), 187–88.

Certain, LK & Kahn, RS (2002). Prevalence, correlates, and trajectory of television viewing among infants and toddlers. *Pediatrics, 109*(4), 634–42.

Chamberlain, L, Wang, Y & Robinson, M (2006). Does children's screen time predict requests for advertised products? *Archives of Pediatrics and Adolescent Medicine, 160*(4).

Dennison, BA, Erb, TA & Jenkins, PL (2002). Television viewing and television in bedroom associated with overweight risk among low-income preschool children. *Pediatrics, 109*(6), 1028–35.

Devlin, L. (2004). Measures taken in New South Wales to address childhood obesity following the NSW Childhood Obesity Summit. *NSW Public Health Bulletin, 15*(4), 68–71.

Dollman, J, Norton, K, Norton, L & Cleland, V (2005). Evidence from secular trends in children's physical activity behaviour. *British Journal of Sports Medicine, 39*(12), 892–97.

Dunstan, DW, Zimmet, PZ, Welborn, T, De Courten, M et al. (2002). The rising prevalence of diabetes and impaired glucose tolerance: the Australian Diabetes and Obesity Lifestyle study. *Diabetes Care, 25*(5), 829–34.

Elias, N & Dunning, E (1986). *Quest for Excitement: Sport and Leisure in the Civilizing Process.* Oxford: Basil Blackwell.

Engeland, A, Bjorge, T, Sogaard, AJ & Tverdal, A (2003). Body mass index in adolescence in relation to total mortality: 32-year follow-up of 227,000 Norwegian boys and girls. *American Journal of Epidemiology, 157*, 517–23.

Foucault, M (1977). *Discipline and Punish: The Birth of the Prison.* London: Allen Lane.

Foucault, M (1984). *The History of Sexuality.* Harmondsworth: Penguin Books.

Francis, LA, Lee, Y & Birch, LL (2003). Parental weight status and girls' television viewing, snacking, and body mass indexes. *Obesity Research, 11*(1), 143–51.

Giammattei, J, Blix, G, Marshak, HH, Wollitzer, AO & Pettitt, DJ (2003). Television watching and soft drink consumption: associations with obesity in 11- to 13-year-old school children. *Archives of*

Pediatrics and Adolescent Medicine, 157(9), 882–86.

Goldberg, ME, Gorn, GJ & Gibson, W (1978). TV messages for snack and breakfast foods: do they influence children's preferences? *Journal of Consumer Research, 5,* 73–81.

Gordon-Larsen, P, McMurray, RG & Popkin, B (2000). Determinants of adolescent physical activity and inactivity patterns. *Pediatrics, 105*(6), E83.

Hancox, RJ, Milne, BJ & Poulton, R (2004). Association between child and adolescent television viewing and adult health: a longitudinal birth cohort study (Abstract). *The Lancet, 364,* 257–62.

Harten, NR & Olds, TS (2004). Patterns of active transport in 11–12 year old Australian children. *Australian and New Zealand Journal of Public Health, 28*(2), 167–72.

Kavanagh, A, Goller, J, King, T, Jolley, D, Crawford, D, Turrell, G (2005). Urban area disadvantage and physical activity: a multilevel study in Melbourne, Australia. *Journal of Epidemiology and Community Health, 59,* doi:10.1136/jech.2005.035931), 934–940.

Lobstein, T, Baur, L & Uauy, R (2004). Obesity in children and young people: a crisis in public health. *Obesity Reviews, 5*(s1), 4–85.

Lumeng, JC, Rahnama, S, Appugliese, D, Kaciroti, N & Bradley, RH (2006). Television exposure and overweight risk in preschoolers. *Archives of Pediatrics and Adolescent Medicine, 160,* 417–22.

Maccoby, E (1951). Television: its impact on school children. *The Public Opinion Quarterly, 15*(3), 421–44.

Magarey, AM, Daniels, LA, et al. (2001). Prevalence of overweight and obesity in Australian children and adolescents: reassessment of 1985 and 1995 data against new standard international definitions. *Medical Journal of Australia, 174,* 561–64.

Mander, J (1978). *Four Arguments for the Elimination of Television.* New York: Quill.

National Health and Medical Research Centre (1997). *Acting on Australia's Weight: A Strategic Plan for the Prevention of Overweight and Obesity.* Canberra: Australian Government Printing Service.

National Obesity Taskforce (2003). *Healthy Weight 2008 — Australia's Future. The National Action Agenda for Children and Young People and Their Families.* Canberra: Commonwealth Department of Health and Ageing. <www.healthyactive.gov.au/docs/healthy_weight08. pdf>.

NSW Department of Health (2003). *Prevention of Obesity in Children and Young People: NSW Government Action Plan 2003–2007.*

Olds, TS, Dollman, J, Ridley, K, Boshoff, K, Hartshorne, S & Kennaugh, S (2004). *Children and Sport.* Adelaide: University of South Australia.

Olds, TS, Ridley, K & Dollman, J (2006). Screenieboppers and extreme screenies: the place of screen time in the time budgets of 10–13-year-old Australian children. *Australian and New Zealand Journal of Public Health, 30*(2), 137–42.

Palmer, P (1986). *The Lively Audience: A Study of Children Around the TV Set*. Sydney: Allen & Unwin.

Parsons, T (1964). *Essays in Sociological Theory*. New York: Free Press.

Parsons, T, Power, C & Manor, O (2005). Physical activity, television viewing and body mass index: a cross-sectional analysis from childhood to adulthood in the 1958 British cohort. *International Journal of Obesity, 29*, 1212–21.

Robotham, J (2006, 22–23 April). Overweight boys at greater risk than girls. *Sydney Morning Herald*, p. 8.

Salmon, J, Campbell, KJ & Crawford, D (2006). Television viewing habits associated with obesity risk factors: a survey of Melbourne schoolchildren. *Medical Journal of Australia, 184*(2), 64–67.

Salmon, J, Timperio, A, Cleland, V & Venn, A (2005). Trends in children's physical activity and weight status in high and low socio-economic status areas of Melbourne, Victoria, 1985–2001. *Australian and New Zealand Journal of Public Health, 29*(4), 337–42.

Salmon, J, Timperio, A, Telford, A, Carver, A & Crawford, D (2005). Association of family environment with children's television viewing and with low level of physical activity. *Obesity Research, 13*, 1939–51.

Sekine, M, Yamagami, T, Handa, K, Saito, T, Nanris, S, Kawaminami, K et al. (2002). A dose-response relationship between short sleeping hours and childhood obesity: results of the Toyama Birth Cohort Study (Abstract). *Child: Care, Health & Development, 28*(2), 163–70.

Skidmore, PML & Yarnel, IJWG (2004). The obesity epidemic: prospects for prevention. *QJM: An International Journal of Medicine, 97*(12), 817–25.

Vandewater, E, Shim, M & Caplovitz, A (2004). Linking obesity and activity level with children's television and video game use. *Journal of Adolescence, 27*(1), 71–85.

Venn, A & Dwyer, T (2005). *Australian Schools Health and Fitness Survey*. Paper presented at the Australian Institute of Science and Technology Convention, Sydney Convention and Exhibition Centre.

Wake, M, Hesketh, K & Waters, E (2003). Television, computer use and body mass index in Australian primary school children. *Journal of Paediatrics and Child Health, 39*(2), 130–34.

Wiecha, JL, Peterson, KE, Ludwig, DS, Kim, J, Sobol, A & Gortmaker, S (2006). When children eat what they watch: impact of television viewing on dietary intake in youth. *Archives of Pediatrics and Adolescent Medicine, 160*, 436–42.

Williams, R (1974). *Television: Technology and Cultural Form*. London: Fontana/Collins.

World Health Organization (ed.) (2000). *Obesity: Preventing and Managing the Global Epidemic*. WHO Technical Series 894. Geneva: WHO.

Wright, C (1975). *Mass Communication: A Sociological Perspective* (2nd edn). New York: Random House.

Wright, C, Parker, L, Lamont, D & Craft, A (2001). Implications of childhood obesity for adult health: findings from thousand families cohort study. *British Medical Journal, 323*, 1280–84.

Sin#5 The car-reliant environment

Australian Bureau of Statistics (2001). Transport Special Article – History of Roads in Australia. *Year Book Australia 2002 (1301.0)* Retrieved 15 October 2003 from <www.abs.gov.au>.

—— (2002). *2001 Census Basic Community Profile and Snapshot*. Canberra: ABS.

—— (2003, 8 April). Driving to Pluto and back: Australians drive 190 billion kilometres (Media Release Cat. No. 9208.0). Retrieved 15 October 2003 from <www.abs.gov.au>.

—— (2005). *Sales of New Motor Vehicles* (Cat. No. 9314.0.55.001). Table 1: New Motor Vehicle Sales by Type, All series. Canberra: ABS.

Austroads (2000). *Road Facts 2000*. Sydney: Austroads Incorporated.

Banwell, C, Dixon, J, Hinde, S & McIntyre, H (2005). Fast and slow food in the fast lane: automobility and the Australian diet. In R Wilk (ed.), *Fast Food/Slow Food: The Cultural Economy of the Global Food System* (vol. 24). California: AltaMira Press.

Banwell, C, Hinde, S, Dixon, J & Sibthorpe, B (2005). Reflections on expert consensus: a case study of the social trends contributing to obesity. *European Journal of Public Health, 15*(6), 564–68.

Beckmann, J (2001). Automobility: a social problem and theoretical concept. *Environment and Planning D: Society and Space, 19*, 593–607.

Bostock, L (2001). Pathways of disadvantage? Walking as a mode of transport among low-income mothers. *Health and Social Care in the Community, 9*(1), 11–18.

Commonwealth Treasurer (2004). Transcript The Hon Peter Costello MP, Treasurer. Doorstop Interview: Wednesday, 21 January 2004 12.15 p.m. Patterson Cheney Holden Ringwood, Melbourne. Retrieved 6 February 2004 from <www.treasurer.gov.au/tsr/content/transcripts/2004/005.asp>.

Davison, G (2004). *Car Wars: How the Car Won our Hearts and Conquered our Cities.* Crows Nest: Allen & Unwin.

Dora, C & Phillips, M (2000). *Transport, Environment and Health.* Copenhagen: World Health Organization Regional Office for Europe.

Dowling, R (2000). Cultures of mothering and car use in suburban Sydney: a preliminary investigation. *Geoforum, 31,* 345–53.

Drugs and Crime Prevention Committee (2005). *Inquiry into Violence Associated with Motor Vehicle Use.* Melbourne: Australian Institute of Criminology. Funded by Parliament of Victoria, Drugs and Crime Prevention Committee.

Fischler, C (1988). Food, self and identity. *Social Science Information, 27,* 275–92.

Frank, L, Andresen, M & Schmid, T (2004). Obesity relationships with community design, physical activity, and time spent in cars. *American Journal of Preventive Medicine, 27*(2), 87–96.

Freund, P & Martin, G (1996). The commodity that is eating the world: the automobile, the environment, and capitalism. *Capitalism, Nature and Socialism, 7*(4), 3–29.

Frumkin, H, Frank, L & Jackson, R (2004). *Urban Sprawl and Public Health: Designing, Planning and Building for Healthy Communities.* Washington: Island Press.

Hamilton, C & Barbato, C (2005). *Who drives 4WDs? (Webpaper).* Canberra: The Australia Institute.

Handy, S, Weston, L & Mokhtarian, PL (2005). Driving by choice or necessity? *Transportation Research Part A: Policy and Practice, 39*(2–3), 183–203.

Heelan, KA, Donnelly, JE, Jacobsen, DJ, Mayo, MS, Washburn, R & Greene, L (2005). Active commuting to and from school and BMI in elementary school children: preliminary data. *Child Care Health and Development, 31*(3), 341–49.

Hinde, S & Dixon, J (2005). Changing the 'obesogenic environment': insights from a cultural economy of car-reliance. *Transportation Research Part D: Transport and Environment, 10*(1), 31–53.

Kavanagh, AM, Goller, JL, King, T, Jolley, D, Crawford, D & Turrell, G (2005). Urban area disadvantage and physical activity: a multilevel study in Melbourne, Australia. *Journal of Epidemiology and Community Health, 59*(11), 934–40.

Kjellstrom, T, van Kerkhoff, L, Bammer, G & McMichael, T (2003). Comparative assessment of transport risks: how it can contribute to health impact assessment of transport policies. *Bulletin of the World Health Organization, 81*(6), 451–57.

Laird, P, Newman, P, Bachels, M & Kenworthy, J (2001). *Back on Track: Rethinking Transport Policy in Australia and New Zealand.* Sydney: UNSW Press.

Mackett, RL, Lucas, L, Paskins, J & Turbin, J (2005). The therapeutic value of children's everyday travel. *Transportation Research Part A: Policy and Practice, 39*(2–3), 205–19.

McMichael, T (2001). *Human Frontiers, Environments and Disease.* Cambridge: Cambridge University Press.

Mason, C (2000a). Healthy people, places and transport. *Health Promotion Journal of Australia, 10*(3), 190–96.

—— (2000b). Transport and health: en route to a healthier Australia? *Medical Journal of Australia, 172*(5), 230–32.

Mathers, C, Vos, T & Stevenson, C (1999). *The Burden of Disease and Injury in Australia.* Canberra: Australian Institute of Health and Welfare.

Mees, P (2000). *A Very Public Solution: Transport in the Dispersed City.* Melbourne: Melbourne University Press.

Miller, D (2001). Driven societies. In D Miller (ed.), *Car Cultures.* Oxford: Berg.

Newman, P (2005). Are we creating a liveable city? Presentation by Prof Peter Newman, NSW Sustainability Commissioner. Retrieved 10 October 2005 from <www.fabian.org.au>.

Paterson, M (2000). Car culture and global environmental politics. *Review of International Studies, 26,* 253–70.

Pikora, T, Giles-Corti, B, Bull, F, Jamrozik, K & Donovan, R (2003). Developing a framework for assessment of the environmental determinants of walking and cycling. *Social Science and Medicine, 56*(8), 1693–1703.

Sheller, M & Urry, J (2000). The city and the car. *International Journal of Urban and Regional Research, 24*(4), 737–57.

Timperio, A, Ball, K, Salmon, J, Roberts, R, Giles-Corti, B, Simmons, D et al. (2006). Personal, family, social, and environmental correlates of active commuting to school. *American Journal of Preventive Medicine, 30*(1), 45–51.

Timperio, A, Crawford, D, Telford, A & Salmon, J (2004). Perceptions about the local neighborhood and walking and cycling among children. *Preventive Medicine, 38*(1), 39–47.

Tudor-Locke, C, Ainsworth, BE, Adair, LS & Popkin, BM (2003). Objective physical activity of Filipino youth stratified for commuting mode to school. *Medicine and Science in Sports and Exercise, 35*(3), 465–71.

Wen, L, Orr, N, Millett, C & Rissel, C (2006). Driving to work and overweight and obesity: findings from the 2003 New South Wales Health Survey, Australia. *International Journal of Obesity, 30*(5), 782–86.

Wollen, P (2002). Introduction. In P Wollen & J Kerr (eds), *Autopia: Cars and Culture* (pp. 10–20). London: Reaktion Books, Ltd.

Sin#6 The marketed environment

Agras, WS, Kraemer, HC, Berkowitz, RI, Korner, AF & Hammer, LD (1987) Does a vigorous feeding style influence early development of adiposity? *Journal of Pediatrics*, *110*(5), 799–804.

Ailhood, G & Guesnet, P (2004). Fatty acid composition of fats is an early determinent of childhood obesity: a short review and an opinion, *Obesity Research*, *5*(21–26).

American Academy of Pediatrics (AAP) (2005). Policy statement: breastfeeding and the use of human milk, *Pediatrics*, *115*(2 February), 496–506.

Arenz, S, Ruckerl, R, Koletzko, B & von Kries, R (2004). Breast-feeding and childhood obesity: a systematic review, *International Journal of Obesity Related Metabolic Disorders*, *28*(10), 1247–56.

Armstrong, W (1939). The infant welfare movement in Australia. *Medical Journal of Australia*, *2*, 641–48.

Australian Bureau of Statistics (1969). *Official Year Book Australia*. Canberra: ABS.

Australian Institute of Health and Welfare (2003). Australia's Welfare 2003 (Cat No. AUS 41). Canberra: AIHW.

Austveg, B & Sundby, J (1995). *Empowerment of Women: The Case of Breastfeeding in Norway*. Oslo: Norwegian Breastfeeding Association.

Baird, J, Fisher, D, Lucas, P, Kleijnen, J, Roberts, H & Law, C (2005). Being big or growing fast: systematic review of size and growth in infancy and later obesity. *British Medical Journal*, *331*(7522), 929.

Baughcum, AE, Burklow, KA, Deeks, CM, Powers, SW & Whitaker, RC (1998). Maternal feeding practices and childhood obesity: a focus group study of low-income mothers. *Archives of Pediatrics and Adolescent Medicine*, *152*(10), 1010–4.

Birch, LL & Fisher, JO (1998). Development of eating behaviors among children and adolescents. *Pediatrics*, *101*(3 Pt 2), 539–49.

Chaloupka, FJ, Jha, P, de Beyer, J & Heller, P (2005). The economics of tobacco control. *Briefing Notes in Economics*, *0*(63), 1–9.

Commonwealth of Australia (2003). *Healthy Weight 2008: Australia's Future: The National Action Agenda for Children, Young People and Their Families*. Canberra.

Dewey, K, Peerson, J, Brown, K, Krebs, N, Michaelsen, K, Persson, L, Salmenpera, L, Whitehead, R & Yeung, D (1995). Growth of breast-fed infants deviates from current reference data: a pooled analysis of US, Canadian, and European data sets. World Health Organization Working Group on Infant Growth. *Pediatrics*, *96*(3), 495–503.

Dewey, KG (2003). Is breastfeeding protective against child obesity? *Journal of Human Lactation*, *19*(1), 9–18.

Dewey, KG, Heinig, MJ & Nommsen, LA (1993). Maternal weight-loss patterns during prolonged lactation. *American Journal of Clinical Nutrition, 58*(2), 162–66.

Dietz, WH (2001). Breastfeeding may help prevent childhood overweight. *Journal of the American Medical Association, 285*(19), 2506–07.

Ebrahim, GJ (1978). *Breast Feeding: The Biological Option*, London: Macmillan.

Enkin, MW, Keirse, MJ, Renfrew, MJ & Neilson, JP (1995). *A Guide to Effective Care in Pregnancy and Childbirth*. Oxford: Oxford University Press.

Featherstone, L (2001). Whose breast is best: Wet nursing in late nineteenth century Australia, *Birth Issues, 11*(2/3), 41–45.

Fomon, SJ, Filmer, LJ, Jr, Thomas, LN, Anderson, TA & Nelson, SE (1975). Influence of formula concentration on caloric intake and growth of normal infants. *Acta Paediatrica Scandinavica, 64*(2), 172–81.

Gabriel, R, Pollard, G, Suleman, G, Coyne, T & Vidgen, H (2005). *Infant and Child Nutrition in Queensland 2003*. Brisbane: Queensland Health.

Gillman, MW, Rifas-Shiman, S, Berkey, C, Frazier, A, Rockett, H, Camargo, C, Field, A & Colditz, G (2006). Breastfeeding and overweight in adolescence. *Epidemiology, 17*(1), 112–14.

Greer, FR & Apple, RD (1991). Physicians, formula companies, and advertising: a historical perspective. *American Journal of Diseases of Children, 145*(3), 282–86.

Hamosh, M (2001). Bioactive factors in human milk. *Pediatric Clinics of North America, 48*(1), 69–86.

Harder, T, Bergmann, R, Kallischnigg, G & Plagemann, A (2005). Duration of breastfeeding and risk of overweight: a meta-analysis. *American Journal of Epidemiology, 162*(5), 397–403.

Hector, D, Webb, K & Lymer, S (2005). *Report on Breastfeeding in NSW 2004 (revised)*. Sydney: NSW Centre for Public Health Nutrition, University of Sydney and NSW Department of Health.

Jutel, A (2001). Does size really matter? weight and values in public health. *Perspectives in Biology and Medicine, 44*(2), 283–96.

Koletzko, B, Agostoni, C, Carlson, SE, Clandinin, T, Hornstra, G, Neuringer, M, Uauy, R, Yamashiro, Y & Willatts, P (2001). Long chain polyunsaturated fatty acids (LC-PUFA) and perinatal development. *Acta Paediatrics Scandinavica, 90*(4), 460–64.

Kramer, MS, Guo, T, Platt, RW, Shapiro, S, Collet, JP, Chalmers, B, Hodnett, E, Sevkovskaya, Z, Dzikovich, I & Vanilovich, I (2002). Breastfeeding and infant growth: biology or bias? *Pediatrics, 110*(2 Pt 1), 343–47.

Lawlor, DA (2005). Infant feeding and components of the metabolic syndrome: findings from the European Youth Heart Study. *Archives of Disease in Childhood, 90*(6), 582–88.

Lucas, A (1991). Programming by early nutrition in man. *Ciba Foundation Symposium, 156,* 38–50; discussion 50–05.

Lucas, A (1998). Programming by early nutrition: an experimental approach. *American Society for Nutritional Sciences,* 128 (2 Supplement), pp. 401S–406S.

Lucas, A (2000). Programming not metabolic imprinting. *American Journal of Clinical Nutrition, 71*(2), 602.

Lucas, A, Bloom, SR & Aynsley-Green, A (1980). Development of gut hormone responses to feeding in neonates. *Archives of Disease in Childhood, 55*(9), 678–82.

Lucas, A, Lucas, PJ & Baum, JD (1979). Pattern of milk flow in breast-fed infants. *Lancet, 2*(8133), 57–58.

Lund-Adams, M & Heywood, P (1995). Breastfeeding in Australia. *World Review of Nutrition and Dietetics, 78,* 75–109.

Lyle, RE, Kincaid, SC, Bryant, JC, Prince, AM & McGehee, RE, Jr (2001). Human milk contains detectable levels of immunoreactive leptin. *Advances in Experimental Medicine and Biology, 501,* 87–92.

McCalman, J (1984). *Struggletown: Public and Private Life in Richmond 1900–1965,* Melbourne: Melbourne University Press.

Martin, RM, Ebrahim, S, Griffin, M, Davey Smith, G, Nicolaides, AN, Georgiou, N, Watson, S, Frankel, S, Holly, JM & Gunnell, D (2005). Breastfeeding and atherosclerosis: intima-media thickness and plaques at 65-year follow-up of the Boyd Orr cohort. *Arteriosclerosis, Thrombosis and Vascular Biology, 25*(7), 1482–88.

Martin, RM, Gunnell, D & Smith, GD (2005). Breastfeeding in infancy and blood pressure in later life: systematic review and meta-analysis. *American Journal of Epidemiology, 161*(1), 15–26.

Mein Smith, P (1988). Truby King in Australia: a revisionist view of reduced infant mortality. *New Zealand Journal of History, 22*(1, April), 23–43.

Mein Smith, P (1997). *Mothers and King Baby: Infant Survival and Welfare in an Imperial World: Australia, 1880–1950.* London: Macmillan.

Minchin, M (1985). *Breastfeeding Matters.* Wendouree, Victoria, and North Sydney, New South Wales: Alma Publications and George Allen & Unwin.

Minchin, M (1998). *Breastfeeding Matters.* Melbourne: Alma Publications.

Mortenson, K (2001). 'Australian Breastfeeding Statistics', Lactation Resource Centre Hot Topics no. 8, Melbourne.

Moynihan, R & Henry, D (2006). The fight against disease mongering: generating knowledge for action. *PLoS Medicine, 3*(4), e191.

National Health and Medical Research Council (NHMRC) (2003). *Dietary Guidelines for Children and Adolescents in Australia Incorporating the Infant Feeding Guidelines for Health Workers*, National Health and Medical Research Council, Canberra, 10 April 2003, NHMRC, Dietary Guidelines for Children and Adolescents in Australia incorporating the Infant Feeding Guidelines for Health Workers, Commonwealth of Australia, 2003 [copy of guidelines on CD or available at <www.nhmrc.gov.au/publications/synopses/dietsyn.htm>].

Ohlin, A & Rossner, S (1990). Maternal body weight development after pregnancy. *International Journal of Obesity*, 14(2), 159–73.

Owen, CG, Martin, RM, Whincup, PH, Smith, GD & Cook, DG (2005). Effect of infant feeding on the risk of obesity across the life course: a quantitative review of published evidence. *Pediatrics*, 115(5), 1367–77.

Plagemann, A & Harder, T (2005). Breast-feeding and the risk of obesity and related metabolic diseases in the child. *Metabolic Syndrome and Related Disorders*, 3(3), 222–32.

Post, JE & Smith, RA (1988). The influence of marketing on infant feeding. In B Winicoff, MA Castle & VH Laukaran (eds), *Feeding Infants in Four Societies: Causes and Consequences of Mothers' Choices*, Population Council/Greenwood Press, New York, 165–86.

Quinn, VJ, Guyon, AB, Schubert, JW, Stone-Jimenez, M, Hainsworth, MD & Martin, LH (2005). Improving breastfeeding practices on a broad scale at the community level: success stories from Africa and Latin America. *Journal of Human Lactation*, 21(3), 345–54.

Ravelli, AC, van der Meulen, JH, Osmond, C, Barker, DJ & Bleker, OP (2000). Infant feeding and adult glucose tolerance, lipid profile, blood pressure, and obesity. *Archives of Disease in Childhood*, 82(3), 248–52.

Reiger, K (2001). *Our Bodies Our Babies*. Melbourne: Melbourne University Press.

Reiger, KM (1985). The Disenchantment of the Home: Modernizing Australian Domestic Life. Melbourne: Oxford University Press.

Reiger, KM (1991). *Family Economy*. Ringwood, Victoria: McPhee Gribble.

Ryan, K & Beresford, RA (1997). The power of support groups: influence on infant feeding trends in New Zealand. *Journal of Human Lactation*, 13(3), 183–90.

Singhal, A, Cole, TJ, Fewtrell, M, Deanfield, J & Lucas, A (2004). Is slower early growth beneficial for long-term cardiovascular health? *Circulation*, 109(9), 1108–13.

Singhal, A, Farooqi, IS, O'Rahilly, S, Cole, TJ, Fewtrell, M & Lucas, A (2002). Early nutrition and leptin concentrations in later life.

American Journal of Clinical Nutrition, 75(6), 993–99.

Siskind, V, Del-Mar, C & Schofield, F (1993). Infant feeding in Queensland, Australia: long term trends. *American Journal of Public Health,* 83(1), 103–06.

Smibert, J (1988). A History of Breastfeeding. *Breastfeeding Review,* 1(12), 14–19.

Sullivan, SA & Birch, LL (1994). Infant dietary experience and acceptance of solid foods. *Pediatrics,* 93(2), 271–77.

Taveras, EM, Scanlon, KS, Birch, L, Rifas-Shiman, SL, Rich-Edwards, JW & Gillman, MW (2004). Association of breastfeeding with maternal control of infant feeding at age 1 year. *Pediatrics,* 114(5), e577–83.

Thorley, V (2002). Maternal dietary advice as an artifact of time and culture: post-World War II Queensland, Australia. *Breastfeeding Review,* 10(1), 25–29.

Thorley, V (2003). Commercial interests and advice on infant history. *Health and History,* 5(1), 65–89.

Truss, W (2004). $2.2 million Australian Government boost for agribusiness. *Press release DAFF04/354WT,* 16 December.

Ventura, A, Savage, J, May, A & Birch, L (2005). Early behavioural, familial and psychosocial predictors of overweight and obesity. In R Tremblay, R Barr & R Peters (eds), *Encyclopedia on Early Childhood Development [online],* Centre of Excellence for Early Childhood Development Montreal, Quebec. Retrieved 18 June 2006 from <www.excellence-earlychildhood.ca/documents/Ventura-Savage-May-BirchANGxp.pdf>.

WHO (1981). 'International Code of Marketing of Breastmilk Substitutes', World Health Organization. Retrieved 12 December 2004 from <www.who.int/nut/documents/code_english.PDF>.

WHO Division of Child Health and Development 1998. *Evidence for the Ten Steps to Successful Breastfeeding,* Geneva: World Health Organization.

Wickes, IG (1953). A history of infant feeding. *Archives of Disease in Childhood,* 28(142), 495–502.

Wolf, JH (2000). The social and medical construction of lactation pathology. *Women's Health,* 30(3), 93–110.

World Health Assembly (Fifty Fourth) (2001). Infant and Young Child Nutrition: Resolution 54.2: Geneva.

World Health Organization (WHO) (2003). Joint WHO/FAO Expert Report on Diet, Nutrition and the Prevention of Chronic Disease. Geneva: WHO.

—— (2006). 'Child growth and development', World Health Organization. Retrieved 18 May 2006 from <www.who.int/nutrition/media_page/en/index.html>.

Sin#7 The environment of competing authorities

Australian Bureau of Statistics (2006a). *National Health Survey: Summary of Results Australia, 2004–05* (Cat No. 4364.0). Canberra: ABS.

—— (2006b). *Sport and Recreation: A Statistical Overview, Australia, 2003* (Cat. No. 4156.0). Canberra: ABS.

Brabazon, T (2000). Time for a change or more of the same? Les Mills and the masculinisation of aerobics. *Sporting Tradition, 17*(1), 102.

Couzin, J (2005). A heavyweight battle over CDC's obesity forecasts. *Science, 308,* 770–71.

Crossley, N (2005). In the gym: motives, meanings and moral careers. *CRESC Working Paper Series Working Paper No. 6.*

Dixon, J (2003). Authority, power and value in contemporary industrial food systems. *International Journal of the Sociology of Agriculture and Food, 11*(1), 31–39.

Dixon, J & Banwell, C (2004). Reembedding trust: unravelling the construction of modern diets. *Critical Public Health, 14*(2), 117–31.

Duff, J (2004). Setting the menu: dietary guidelines, corporate interests, and nutrition policy. In J Germov & L Williams (eds), *A Sociology of Food and Nutrition: The Social Appetite* (2nd edn, pp. 148–69). Melbourne: Oxford University Press.

Eccleston, R (2006). Fat fighters. *Weekend Australian Magazine,* 20–23.

Elinder, LS (2005). Obesity, hunger, and agriculture: the damaging role of subsidies. *British Medical Journal, 331*(7528), 1333–36.

Fischler, C (1988). Food, self and identity. *Social Science Information, 27*(2), 275–92.

Frew, M & McGillivray, D (2005). Health clubs and body politics: aesthetics and the quest for physical capital. *Leisure Studies, 24*(2).

Frey, J & Eitzen, DS (1991). Sport and society. *Annual Review of Sociology, 17,* 503–22.

Gabriel, Y & Lang, T (1995). *The Unmanageable Consumer.* London: Sage.

Glassner, B (1989). Fitness and the postmodern self. *Journal of Health and Social Behavior, 30,* 180–91.

Harris, J & Marandi, E (2002). The gendered dynamics of relationship marketing: an initial discussion of the health and fitness industry. *Managing Leisure 7,* 194–200.

Hull, W (1962). The public control of broadcasting: the Canadian and Australian experiences. *The Canadian Journal of Economics and Political Science, 28*(1), 114–26.

Humphery, K (1998). *Shelf Life: Supermarkets and the Changing Culture of Consumption.* Cambridge, UK: Cambridge University Press.

Jaher, F (1977). Sport in modern America. *Reviews in American History, 5*(1), 1–7.

Katz, DL (2005). Competing dietary claims for weight loss: finding the forest through truculent trees. *Annual Review of Public Health, 26*, 61–88.

Kegan, E & Morse, M (1988). The body electronic: aerobic exercise on video: a women's search for empowerment and self-transformation. *TDR, 32*(4), 164–80.

Kersh, R & Morone, J (2002). The politics of obesity: seven steps to government action. *Health Affairs, 21*(6), 142–50.

Kirk, D & Macdonald, D (1998). The physical activity profession in process: unity, diversity and the Australian Council for Health, Physical Education and Recreation, 1970–1997. *Sporting Traditions, 15*(1), 3–24.

Lang, T, Rayner, G & Kaelin, E (2006). *The Food Industry, Diet, Physical Activity and Health: A Review of Reported Commitments and Practice of 25 of the World's Largest Food Companies.* London: City University.

Lawrence, M & Germov, J (2004). Future food: the politics of functional foods and health claims. In J Germov & L Williams (eds), *A Sociology of Food and Nutrition: The Social Appetite* (2nd edn, pp. 119–47). Melbourne: Oxford University Press.

McDonald, JT & Kennedy, S (2005). Is migration to Canada associated with unhealthy weight gain? Overweight and obesity among Canada's immigrants. *Social Science and Medicine, 61*(12), 2469–81.

McKay, J (1986). Hegemony, the state and Australian sport. In G Lawrence & D Rowe (eds), *Power Play: Essays in the Sociology of Australian Sport* (pp. 115–35). Sydney: Hale & Iremonger.

Nestle, M (2002). *Food Politics.* Berkeley: University of California Press.

Papadaki, A & Scott, JA (2002). The impact on eating habits of temporary translocation from a Mediterranean to a Northern European environment. *European Journal of Clinical Nutrition, 56*, 455–61.

Philips, J & Drummond, M (2001). An investigation into the body image perception, body satisfaction and exercise expectations of male fitness leaders: implications for professional practice. *Leisure Studies, 20*, 95–105.

Pileggi, MS & Patton, C (2003). Introduction: Bourdieu and cultural studies. *Cultural Studies, 17*(3/4), 313–25.

Popkin, B (1993). Nutritional patterns and transitions. *Population Development Review, 19*, 138–57.

Powles, J (2001). Commentary: Mediterranean paradoxes continue to provoke. *International Journal of Epidemiology, 30*, 1076–77.

Rader, B (1991). The quest for self-sufficiency and the new strenuosity: reflections on the strenuous life of the 1970s and the 1980s. *Journal of Sport History, 18*(2), 255–66.

Rozin, P (2005). The meaning of food in our lives: a cross-cultural perspective on eating and well-being. *Journal of Nutrition Education and Behavior, 37*(Supplement 2), S107–S112.

Rozin, P, Fischler, C, Imada, S, Sarubin, A & Wrzensniewski, A (1999). Attitudes to food and the role of food in life in the U.S.A, Japan, Flemish Belgium and France: possible implications for the diet–health debate. *Appetite, 33*, 163–80.

Rozin, P, Kabnick, K, Pete, E, Fischler, C & Shields, C (2003). The ecology of eating: smaller portion sizes in France than in the United States help explain the French paradox. *Psychological Science, 14*(5), 450–54.

Sassatelli, R (2001). The commercialization of discipline: keep-fit culture and its values. *Journal of Modern Italian Studies, 5*(3), 396–411.

Simon, M (2005). Junk food's health crusade: how Ronald McDonald became a health ambassador, and other stories. *Multinational Monitor, 26*(3–4).

Stewart, B (1986). Sport as big business. In G Lawrence & D Rowe (eds), *Power Play: Essays in the Sociology of Australian Sport* (pp. 64–84). Sydney: Hale & Iremonger.

Sundquist, J & Winkleby, M (2000). Country of birth, acculturation status and abdominal obesity in a national sample of Mexican-American women and men. *International Journal of Epidemiology, 29*(3), 470–77.

Willcox, J (2006). The couch-potato games. *Sydney Morning Herald*, p. 13.

Unequal society, unhealthy weight: The social distribution of obesity

Australian Bureau of Statistics (2000). *Apparent Consumption of Foodstuffs in Australia 1997–1998 and 1998–1999.* Canberra: ABS.

Ball, K & Crawford, D (2005). Socioeconomic status and weight change in adults: a review. *Social Science and Medicine, 60*(9), 1987–2010.

Ball, K, Crawford, D, Ireland, P & Hodge, A (2002). Patterns and demographic predictors of 5-year weight change in a multi-ethnic cohort of men and women in Australia. *Public Health Nutrition, 6*(3), 269–80.

Ball, K, Mishra, G & Crawford, D (2002). Which aspects of socioeconomic status are related to obesity among men and women? *International Journal of Obesity, 26*(4), 559–65.

Beer-Borst, S, Morabia, A, Hercberg, S, Vitek, O, Bernstein, MS,

Galan, P et al. (2000). Obesity and other health determinants across Europe: The EURALIM Project. *Journal of Epidemiology and Community Health, 5*(4), 424–30.

Blane, D (2006). Commentary: the place in life course research of validated measures of socioeconomic position. *International Journal of Epidemiology, 35*(1), 139–40.

Booth, M, Chey, T, Wake, M, Norton, K, Hesketh, K, Dollman, J et al. (2003). Change in the prevalence of overweight and obesity among young Australians, 1969–1997. *American Journal of Clinical Nutrition, 77*, 29–36.

Burton, P & Phipps, S (2004). *Families, Time and Money in Canada, Germany, Sweden, the United Kingdom and the United States.* Halifax, Nova Scotia: Department of Economics, Dalhousie University.

Calle, EE, Thun, MJ, Petrelli, JM, Rodriguez, C & Heath, CW (1999). Body-mass index and mortality in a prospective cohort of U.S. adults. *New England Journal of Medicine, 341*(15), 1097–105.

Chang, V & Lauderdale, D (2005). Income disparities in body mass index and obesity in the United States, 1971–2002. *Archives of International Medicine, 165*, 2122–28.

Choi, BCK, Hunter, DJ, Tsou, W & Sainsbury, P (2005). Diseases of comfort: primary cause of death in the 22nd century. *Journal of Epidemiology and Community Health, 59*(12), 1030–34.

Cutler, DM, Glaeser, EL & Shapiro, JM (2003). Why have Americans become more obese? *Journal of Economic Perspectives, 17*(3), 93–118.

Dengler R, Roberts H & Rushton L (1997). Lifestyle surveys: the complete answer? *Journal of Epidemiology and Community Health, 51*, 46–51.

Dowler, E (1997). Budgeting for food on a low-income in the UK: the case of lone parent families. *Food Policy, 22*(5), 405–17.

Drewnowski, A & Specter, S (2004). Poverty and obesity: the role of energy density and energy costs. *American Journal of Clinical Nutrition, 79*(1), 6–16.

Eckersley, R (2001). Losing the battle of the bulge: causes and consequences of increasing obesity. *Medical Journal of Australia, 174*(4 June), 590–92.

Friel, S, Newell, J & Kelleher, C (2005). Who eats four or more servings of fruit and vegetables per day? Multivariate classification tree analysis of data from the 1998 Survey of Lifestyle, Attitudes and Nutrition in the Republic of Ireland. *Public Health Nutrition, 8*(2), 159–69.

Friel, S, Walsh, O & McCarthy, D (accepted May 2006). The irony of a rich country: issues of access and availability of healthy food in the Republic of Ireland. *Journal of Epidemiology and Community Health.*

Galobardes, B, Shaw, M, Lawlor, DA, Lynch, JW & vey Smith, G (2006). Indicators of socioeconomic position (part 1). *Journal of Epidemiology and Community Health, 60*(1), 7–12.

Gordon-Larsen, P, Adair, LS & Popkin, BM (2003). The relationship of ethnicity, socioeconomic factors, and overweight in U.S. adolescents. *Obesity Research, 11*(1), 121–29.

Graham, H (2004). Social determinants and their unequal distribution: clarifying policy understandings. *The Milbank Quarterly, 82*(1), 101–24.

Haraldsdottir, J (1991). *Dietary Surveys and the Use of their Results.* Copenhagen: World Health Organization.

Krieger, N, Williams, D & Moss, N (1997). Measuring social class in US public health research: concepts, methodologies, and guidelines. *Annual. Review Public Health, 18*, 341–78.

Lallukka, T, Laaksonen, M, Martikainen, P, Sarlio-Lahteenkorva, S & Lahelma, E (2005). Psychosocial working conditions and weight gain among employees. *29*(8), 909–15.

Langenberg, C, Hardy, R, Kuh, D, Brunner, E & Wadsworth, M (2003). Central and total obesity in middle aged men and women in relation to lifetime socioeconomic status: evidence from a national birth cohort. *Journal of Epidemiology and Community Health, 57*(10), 816–22.

Loureiro, M & Nayga, R (2005). *Obesity Rates in OECD Countries: An International Perspective.* Paper presented at the EAAE XI Congress, Copenhagen.

Manor O, Matthews S & Power C (1997). Comparing measures of health inequality. *Social Science and Medicine, 45*(5), 761–71.

Mathers, C, Vos, T & Stevenson, C (1999). *The Burden of Disease and Injury in Australia.* Canberra: Australian Institute of Health and Welfare.

Mitra, A (2001). Effects of physical attributes on the wages of males and females. *Applied Economics Letters, 8*(11), 731–35.

Molarius, A, Seidell, J, Sans, S, Tuomilehto, J & Kuulasmaa, K (2000). Educational level, relative body weight, and changes in their association over 10 years: an international perspective from the WHO MONICA Project. *American Journal of Public Health, 90*(8), 1260–68.

Morris, J, Donkin, A, Wonderling, D, Wilkinson, P & Dowler, E (2000). A minimum income for healthy living. *Journal of Epidemiology and Community Health, 54*, 885–89.

Mummery, WK, Schofield, GM, Steele, R, Eakin, EG & Brown, WJ (2005). Occupational sitting time and overweight and obesity in Australian workers. *American Journal of Preventive Medicine, 29*(2), 91–97.

Offer, A (1998). *Epidemics of Abundance: Overeating and Slimming in the USA and Britain Since the 1950s.* Nuffield College: University of Oxford.

Power, C & Matthews, C (1997). Origins of health inequalities in a national population sample. *The Lancet, 35,* 1584–89.

Proper, KI, Cerin, E, Brown, WJ & Owen, N (2006). Sitting time and socioeconomic differences in overweight and obesity. *International Journal of Obesity, International Journal of Obesity advance online publication, 25 April 2006,* doi:10.1038/sj.ijo.0803357.

Rosenbaum, S (1988). 100 years of heights and weights. *Journal of the Royal Statistical Society: Series A (Statistics and Society), 151*(2), 276–309.

Rychetnik, L, Webb, K, Story, L & Katz, T (2003). *Food Security Options Paper: A Planning Framework and Menu of Options for Policy and Practice Interventions.* Sydney: NSW Centre for Public Health Nutrition.

Salmon, J, Owen, N, Bauman, A, Schmitz, MKH & Booth, M (2000). Leisure-time, occupational, and household physical activity among professional, skilled, and less-skilled workers and homemakers. *Preventive Medicine, 30*(3), 191–99.

Seidell, J (2000). Obesity, insulin resistance and diabetes: a worldwide epidemic. *British Journal of Nutrition, 83*(1), 5–8.

Seidell, J (2005). Epidemiology of obesity. *Seminars in Vascular Medicine, 5*(1), 3–14.

Shaw, M, Dorling, D, Gordon, D & Davey-Smith, G (1999). *The Widening Gap: Health Inequalities and Policy in Britain.* Bristol: The Policy Press.

Sobal, J & Stunkard, AJ (1989). Socioeconomic status and obesity: a review of the literature. *Psychological Bulletin, 105*(2), 260–75.

Turrell, G & Najman, J (1995). Collecting food related data from low socioeconomic groups: how adequate are our current research designs? *Australian Journal of Public Health, 19*(4), 410–16.

Turrell, G, Patterson, C, Oldenburg, B, Gould, T & Roy, M (2002). The socio-economic patterning of survey participation and non-response error in a multilevel study of food purchasing behaviour: area- and individual-level characteristics. *Public Health Nutrition, 6*(2), 181–89.

Turrell G, Stanley L, de Looper M & Oldenburg B (2006). *Health Inequalities in Australia: Morbidity, Health Behaviours, Risk Factors and Health Service Use March 2006*: Queensland University of Technology and the Australian Institute of Health and Welfare.

Wardle, J & Griffith, J (2001). Socioeconomic status and weight control practices in British adults. *Journal of Epidemiology and Community Health, 55*(3), 185–90.

Wardle, J, Waller, J & Jarvis, M. J (2002). Sex differences in the association of socioeconomic status with obesity. *American Journal of Public Health, 92*(8), 1299–1304.

Woodward, D, Drager, N, Beaglehole, R & Lipson, D (2001). Globalization and health: a framework for analysis and action. *Bulletin of the World Health Organization, 79,* 875–81.

Yu, Z, Nissinen, A, Vartiainen, E, Song, G, Guo, Z, Zheng, G et al. (2000). Associations between socioeconomic status and cardiovascular risk factors in an urban population in China. *Bulletin of the World Health Organization, 78*(11), 1296–1305.

Zagorsky, JL (2005). Health and wealth: the late-20th century obesity epidemic in the U.S. *Economics & Human Biology, 3*(2), 296–313.

Zweiniger-Bargielowska, I (2005). The culture of the abdomen: obesity and reducing in Britain, circa 1900–1939. *Journal of British Studies, 44*(2), 239–73.

Conclusion

Abelson, P & Taylor, R (2001). Programs to reduce Coronary Heart Disease. In P Abelson (ed.), *Return of Investment in Public Health* (pp. 33–49). Canberra: Department of Health and Ageing.

Australian Bureau of Statistics (2006). *National Health Survey: Summary of Results Australia, 2004–05* (Cat. No. 4364.0). Canberra: ABS.

Ball, K & Crawford, D (2005). Socioeconomic status and weight change in adults: a review. *Social Science and Medicine, 60*(9), 1987–2010.

Banwell, C, Dixon, J, Hinde, S & McIntyre, H (2006). Fast and slow food in the fast lane: automobility and the Australian diet. In R Wilk (ed.), *Fast Food/Slow Food: The Economic Anthropology of the Global Food System* (vol. 24). California: AltaMira Press.

Bauman, Z (2001). Cultural variety or variety of culture. In S Malesevic & M Haugaard (eds), *Making Sense of Collectivity: Identity, Nationalism and Globalisation* (pp. 167–80). London: Pluto Press.

Bennett, T & Silva, E (2006). Introduction. Cultural capital and inequality: policy issues and context. *Cultural Trends, 15,* 87–106.

Bourdieu, P (1984). *Distinction: A Social Critique of the Judgement of Taste.* London: Routledge.

Brownson, R, Haire-Joshu, D & Luke, D (2006). Shaping the context of health: a review of environmental and policy approaches in the prevention of chronic diseases. *Annual Review of Public Health, 27,* 341–70.

Campos, P (2004). *The Obesity Myth: Why America's Obsession with Weight is Hazardous to Your Health.* New York: Gotham Books.

Centers for Disease Control and Prevention (CDCP) (2005). *Public Health Strategies for Preventing and Controlling Overweight and Obesity in School and Worksite Settings: A Report on Recommendations of the Taskforce on Community Preventive Services* (No. MMWR 2005:54 (No. RR-10)). Atlanta: CDCP.

Clarke, J (2004). *Creating Citizen-consumers: The Trajectory of an Identity.* Paper prepared for CASCA Annual Conference, London, Ontario, 5–9 May 2004.

Crossley, N (2004). Fat is a sociological issue: obesity rates in late modern, 'body-conscious' societies. *Social Theory & Health, 2*(3), 222–53.

Crotty, P (1995). *Good nutrition? Fact and Fashion in Dietary Advice.* Sydney: Allen & Unwin.

Dixon, J, Banwell, C & Hinde, S (2006, May 25–26). *Cities, Consumption and Health.* Paper presented at the Urbanism, Environment and Health, Fenner Conference 2006, Canberra.

Dunstan, DW, Zimmet, PZ, Welborn, T, De Courten, M et al. (2002). The rising prevalence of diabetes and impaired glucose tolerance: the Australian Diabetes and Obesity Lifestyle study. *Diabetes Care, 25*(5), 829–34.

Elchardus, M (1991). Flexible men and women. The changing temporal organization of work and culture: an empirical analysis. *Social Science Information, 30*(4), 701–25.

Elchardus, M (1994). In praise of rigidity: on temporal and cultural flexibility. *Informations Sur les Sciences Sociales, 33*(3), 459–77.

Emmison, M (2003). Social class and cultural mobility: Reconfiguring the cultural omnivore thesis. *Journal of Sociology, 39*(3), 211–30.

Fernandez-Armesto, F (2001). *Food: A History.* London: Macmillan.

Gard, M & Wright, J (2005). *The Obesity Epidemic: Science, Morality and Ideology.* London: Routledge.

Gittens, R (2004, 28 July). Why are we losing the battle against time? *The Age,* p. 13.

Goudsblom, J & Mennell, S (eds) (1980). *The Elias Reader.* Oxford: Blackwell.

Hawkes, C (2006). Uneven dietary development: linking the policies and processes of globalization with the nutrition transition, obesity and diet-related chronic diseases. *Globalization and Health, 2*(4), 1–18.

Holtgrave, D & Crosby, R (2006). Is social capital a protective factor against obesity and diabetes? Findings from an exploratory study. *Annual Epidemiology, 16,* 406–08.

Hunt, K & Emslie, C (2001). Commentary: the prevention paradox in lay epidemiology: Rose revisited. *International Journal of Epidemiology, 39,* 442–46.

Jain, A (2005). Treating obesity in individuals and populations. *British Medical Journal 331*, 1387–90.

Jutel, A (2001). Does size really matter? weight and values in public health. *Perspectives in Biology and Medicine, 44*(2), 283–96.

Katz, DL (2005). Competing Dietary Claims for Weight Loss: Finding the forest through truculent trees. *Annual Review of Public Health, 26*, 61–88.

Kersh, R & Morone, J (2002). How the personal becomes political: prohibitions, public health, and obesity. *Studies in American Political Development, 16*, 162–75.

Kumaniyika, S, Jeffery, R, Morabia, A, Ritenbaugh, C & Antipatis, V (2002). Obesity prevention: the case for action. *International Journal of Obesity, 26*, 425–36.

Mackenbach, J (2006). *Health Inequalities: Europe in Profile*. Rotterdam: Erasmus Medical Center.

National Board of Health (2003). *National Action Plan Against Obesity. Recommendations and Perspectives*. Copenhagen: Center for Health Promotion and Prevention, Denmark National Board of Health.

National Health and Medical Research Centre (NHMRC) (1997). *Acting on Australia's Weight: A Strategic Plan for the Prevention of Overweight and Obesity*. Canberra: National Health and Medical Research Centre.

National Heart Foundation of Australia (NHFA) (2003). *Detailed Review of Intervention Studies: How Do We Best Address the Issues of Overweight, Obesity and Cardiovascular Disease?* Melbourne: NHFA.

Newman, P (2006, May 25–26). *Health, Anti-urbanism and Public Policy*. Paper presented at the Urbanism, Environment and Health, Fenner Conference 2006, Canberra.

Powles, J (2001). Healthier progress: historical perspectives on the social determinants of health. In R Eckersley, J Dixon & R Douglas (eds), *The Social Origins of Health and Well-being* (pp. 1–24). Cambridge: Cambridge University Press.

Raine, K (2004). *Overweight and Obesity in Canada: A Population Health Perspective*. Ottowa: Canadian Institute for Health Information.

Santich, B (1995). *What the Doctors Ordered: 150 Years of Dietary Advice*. Melbourne: Hyland House.

Sindall, C, Wright, J & O'Dea, K (1994). Food production, human nutrition and the impact of health messages: a public health perspective. *Proceedings of the Nutrition Society of Australia, 18*, 156–66.

Sobal, J (2001). Commentary: globalization and the epidemiology of obesity. *International Journal of Obesity, 30*, 1136–37.

Strazdins, L (2006, May 25–26). *Designs of the Time: Work, Families and*

Sustainable Cities. Paper presented at the Urbanism, Environment and Health, Fenner Conference 2006, Canberra.

Swinburn, B, Gill, T & Kumanyika, S (2005). Obesity prevention: a proposed framework for translating evidence into action. *Obesity Reviews*, 6(1), 23–33.

Tsai, A & Wadden, T (2005). Systematic review: an evaluation of major commercial weight loss programs in the United States. *Annual of Internal Medicine*, 142(1), 56–66.

Tyrell, I (1999). *Deadly Enemies: Tobacco and its Opponents in Australia*. Sydney: UNSW Press.

Williams, S (1995). Theorising class, health and lifestyles: can Bourdieu help us? *Sociology* of *Health and Illness*, 17(5), 577–604.

World Health Organization (WHO) (2000). *Obesity: Preventing and Managing the Global Epidemic. Report of a WHO Consultation on Obesity* (No. WHO Technical Report Series 894). Geneva: WHO.

INDEX

lay 184, 187

4WDs 95–6
family diet 52–3, 66
family eating patterns 51–3
feeding behaviours 105–7
female labour market trends 119–21
Fischler, Claude 127–8
fitness industry
    aerobics 72, 133–4, 136
    authorities 133–6
    programs 16, 134, 141
    personal trainers 16,
        37, 131, 135–6
    in Scotland 135
    self-empowerment 133–4
Fonda, Jane 133–4
food
    consumption 10, 13, 14, 27,
        47, 86, 90, 96, 126–7
    labelling 28, 103, 123
    preferences 52, 105–6
    service sector 14
    unhealthy 51, 55, 63
formula 18, 104, 106, 111–12,
    113, 116–17, 118, 123
fragmentation of waking
    hours 40–1
France
    childhood obesity 15, 50, 144, 146
    experts 50
fussy eaters 50

gender 153, 154, 158–61, 166–7
genetic theories of obesity 2, 8, 10
'Get Moving' campaign 66–7
globalisation 40, 174
goods and services 14,
    21, 22–5, 39, 178, 185
government policy see public policy
greenhouse gas emissions
    31, 33, 82, 86

health and fitness industry
    see fitness industry
health consequences 85–7
health effects
    of time pressure 43–5
health inequalities 149–51, 175, 184
    social factors 161–6

health issues 3, 4–6, 46, 69, 110,
    150, 153, 158, 161, 173, 179, 184
health literature reports of
    childhood obesity 67–9
health professionals 18, 66,
    110, 112, 115, 123, 124
    direct advertising to 116
healthy eating 16, 51–2, 53,
    55, 105, 128, 147, 164, 177
healthy weight 36, 45, 56, 61,
    162–3, 169, 173, 177, 179
    gain 110–11
heart disease 4, 43, 74, 87,
    103, 106, 142, 180
high energy foods 3,
    36, 52, 73–4, 100
high income families 55,
    76, 156, 158, 160, 167
hospitals 103, 113–15, 116, 123, 130
household production 24–5
human metabolism 10, 106–7
hunter-gatherers 9

income 158–61
    as an indicator 158, 159, 165
income families
    high 55, 76, 156, 158, 160, 167
    low 5, 41, 61–2, 76, 78,
        152, 156, 160, 174
Indigenous Australians 18, 156–7
indirect marketing 132
individual choice 31–4
infant feeding practices 16, 101–25
    age-weight charts 110–11
    artificial feeding 103–4,
        106, 110, 114, 116, 122–4
    and commercial infant
        foods 111–12
    conclusion 122–5
    feeding behaviours 105–7
    female labour market
        trends 119–21
    and healthy weight gain 110–11
    market share competition 112–13
    mass marketing 116–19
    and the medical
        profession 109–10
    nutrition 103–5
    'scientific' maternity care
        services 113–15